LA PARTERA

LA PARTERA

STORY OF A MIDWIFE

FRAN LEEPER BUSS

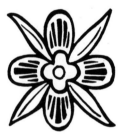

The University of Michigan Press
Ann Arbor

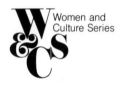

Women and
Culture Series

Library of Congress Cataloging in Publication Data

Buss, Fran Leeper, 1942–
   La partera.

   Bibliography: p.
   1. Maternal health services—New Mexico—San Miguel Co. 2. Aragón,
Jesusita, 1908– 3. Midwives—New Mexico—San Miguel Co.—Bibliog-
raphy. 4. San Miguel Co., N.M.—Social life and customs. I. Title.
RG961.N6B87 1980   362.1'982   80–11784
ISBN 0–472–09322–3
ISBN 0–472–06322–7 (pbk.)

To David, Kimberly, Lisa,
and Jim

WITHDRAWN

Preface

MY HUSBAND, DAVID, our three children, and I moved to northeastern New Mexico in 1975. David and I are both United Church of Christ ministers, and we went there to share a position in an ecumenical campus-community ministry in the town of Las Vegas. I had been involved with women's issues for a number of years and was struck by the strength and independence of many of the older women in the community, and gradually I began to learn the details of their stories.

Throughout the book, the term Hispanic refers to people coming from a Spanish-speaking background, while the term Anglo refers to people coming from the dominant, English-speaking culture of the United States.

I met Jesusita Aragón, the last of the traditional, Hispanic midwives in the area, through several women who had babies with her. It was through them that I first learned some of her history. I knew immediately she had a story worth telling, and Jesusita was eager to tell it.

Jesusita and I began to work on this book in 1976, and our work together continued despite the fact that my family and I moved to Wisconsin. In order to finish the book I returned to New Mexico several times to do research, and Jesusita and I shared countless long distance phone calls.

I also met Edith Rackley through my work in New Mexico. She is a retired public health worker who was one of the first Anglo health care givers to work in the Hispanic villages of the area. She helped me immeasurably by giving me details of the important role of the traditional midwives and the early public health workers in the area. I consider myself fortunate to have been involved in the lives of Jesusita, her family and friends, and the public health workers who were so helpful to me. I have marveled at the warmth and openness of the women in this book, and I have been deeply impressed by their dedication to their work and to each other.

I specifically wish to thank David, Kimberly, Lisa, and Jim for their love and support throughout this project, and, in addition to Jesusita herself, I want to thank Julia Gurulé, Edith Rackley, Dr. Edith Millican, Helen O'Brien, and Anne Fox for their contributions. I also wish to thank those who allowed me to photograph them, Steven Oppenheimer and Paul Pearlman for the use of several of their photographs, Lauri Ahlman for his help in reproducing the photographs, and Pat Shibles for her typing and general assistance.

Contents

Introduction

SHE HAD LIVED AND worked in the canyons and plains since her early childhood, taking the place of the oldest son in the family because her father had no son from his first marriage. She had always worked hard, but after she was forced to leave school at the end of the eighth grade, she herded the sheep and goats full time, leaving on horseback in the early morning, driving them to the canyon to graze throughout the day, and then returning them to the corral again in the evening.

Her work, however, did have a seasonal rhythm. In the spring, in addition to the herding, she helped plant the fields, following along behind the team of three horses with the hand-guided wooden plow, working her way through the dry and rocky soil. In the summer she sheared sheep with the men and sometimes drove the wool to market, and in the fall she helped harvest the food and prepare it for storage through the winter.

Throughout the year, after work in the evenings, she would take off her shoes, wash her feet, close her eyes, and sit on the floor with her back against the wall and rest.

A number of years passed in this way between the time she left school and her "time of troubles." During those long years of hard work she learned the skills of subsistence farming and ranching and how to personally bear the many hours of daily labor. Also, during those years, she learned from her grandmother the beginning skills of midwifery and healing.

The young woman, an Hispanic New Mexican named Jesusita Aragón, is seventy now and has delivered over twelve thousand infants. This is primarily her story, but the telling of her story involves glimpses into the lives of hundreds of women, women whose lives were lived under harsh conditions of poverty and represented an heroic ability to endure. The land and weather have been daily participants in the women's stories. The majority of the women worked outside constantly; many survived on small-scale ranching and nearly subsistence farming. Because of its isolation, the region in which they lived was nearly a frontier just a few decades ago, and these women lived the strenuous lives usually associated with an earlier period in our history.

The land of northeastern New Mexico is culturally and geographically quite different from the rest of the United States. It is an area of orange, pink, and rust colored mountains covered by vast acres of green pine, with blue spruce and fir in the higher, moist areas and scrub pine and piñon in the lower, drier regions. Its altitude is high, sixty-four hundred feet at the base of the mountains, and consequently there is snow in the winter and coldness, but through all the seasons the weather is dominated by striking turquoise skies and a brilliant, penetrating sun. There are winds throughout the year, especially in the spring. When the rains come, primarily as afternoon thunder showers in the summer, much of the red earth becomes caked with mud. This mud is the basic ingredient of *adobe*, the primary building material of the region.

The mountains descend suddenly in the East and become stretches of plains, the *llanos*, as they are called by those who live there. The plains are vast, raw, dry lands, cut through by canyons and *arroyos*. In the past these plains were great fields of grama grass, but in the last decades they have become increasingly arid and desertlike. Now much of the grass has given away to sagebrush; yet still, there is a vastness and stark beauty in the area.

When I lived in New Mexico I drove alone onto the plains,

and within a few minutes I was miles away from another person, alone with only the sounds of the wind and the shifting rays and shadows of the sun. The isolation possible in this part of New Mexico is intense, and from almost any point I could see immense distances to the grey blue mountains on the horizons.

In many ways northeastern New Mexico has also been culturally isolated from the rest of the country. Until the last few decades the Spanish-American village culture of this area was relatively untouched by the urbanization and industrialization taking place in the rest of the United States. For centuries the villages of this area held tenaciously to their own traditions and values, and Spanish has remained their mother tongue.[1]

The basic ancestors of these villagers were the early Iberian colonizers who moved into New Mexico through Mexico in the late seventeenth and early eighteenth centuries. These colonizers founded villages that were isolated from other European groups for almost three centuries, although they established relationships with the Pueblo Indian communities in the area and traded directly with Mexico. Eventually these Spanish-speaking villages developed a distinctive rural culture.[2]

The culture of the mountain villages included shared land, extended family systems that were strongly patriarchal, leadership by the village *patrón*, and the strong influence of folk Catholicism, a Catholicism revolving around the worship of family and village saints.

The culture of the villages of the eastern plains tended to be organized somewhat differently from the mountain villages. They were more loosely formed, with more private land owning and large herds that were grazed on the vast grasslands. These villages were gathering places for the *vaqueros*, the ranchers and their families. Still, the patriarchal family and Catholicism were basic to these villages.[3]

The last fifty years, however, has seen the gradual breakup of these isolated, largely self-sufficient mountain and plains villages. The depression and droughts of the 1930s and beyond deepened the poverty and harsh struggle for existence that had characterized so many lives and forced large numbers of village people to seek government economic assistance.[4]

Increasing numbers of Anglos moved into the area and much of the political and economic control passed into their hands. Numbers of people left the villages and moved into towns. The droughts especially affected the plains, and many of the ranching families and communities simply passed away. Today the back roads of the mountains and plains frequently reveal small, largely abandoned brown and rust adobe villages. A number of the old people, and some of the very young, remain in these villages, but most of the young adults have left to find work elsewhere.

The largest town in this immediate region is Las Vegas, "the meadows"; not Las Vegas, Nevada, as people quickly point out, but "the other Las Vegas." It is the seat of San Miguel County, a largely rural county which straddles the forested mountains, the foothills, and the plains. It is one of the poorest counties in the nation. In 1974 San Miguel County's per capita income was $2,786[5] while the national per capita income was $4,595[6] and in 1977, 24 percent of its families qualified for the food stamp program.[7]

The town, located at the base of the foothills, is cut by the narrow Gallinas River, the "Chicken River," named for the prairie hens and other wild fowl originally living in the meadows.[8] The Gallinas was formerly a good-sized mountain stream, descending to the plains at Las Vegas, but now, because of extensive upstream irrigation, it is often no more than two feet wide and a foot or so deep. Still, it divides the town in half and clearly separates west Las Vegas from east Las Vegas.[9]

The overwhelming majority of west Las Vegas's people are Hispanic New Mexicans. Its many unpaved roads and adobe homes with peaked tin roofs cause it to resemble a large village in northern New Mexico. The town is focused around a plaza which originally was the location of the Catholic church, Our Lady of Sorrows. The church is now in another location. The name of the church refers to *Nuestra Señora de los Dolores*, the grieving mother of Christ frequently turned to for support by the residents of the area.

West Las Vegas, as a whole, has lost much of its economic

vigor and has lived for decades with little growth and high unemployment. However, it is still the home of many of the original founding families, even though young members of these families often migrate to Denver, Albuquerque, or California in search of work and only return for visits.

Jesusita's story involves an understanding of the pre-Anglo, folk medical system that met the health and emotional needs of the Spanish speaking mountains and plains villages. This system was practiced by primarily female folk healers called *curanderas*, or *curanderos* if male.[10] It had been brought originally with settlers from Mexico and, consequently, had much in common with other indigenous Hispanic health care systems.[11]

These Hispanic health care systems stressed the important harmonious relationship between the natural and the supernatural when dealing with human health needs. In addition, the curanderas believed that their ability to cure was a blessing given them by God, an ability they were required to use in the service of others. For these reasons, many of the curanderas' treatments of illnesses and physical misfortunes involved both specifically medical treatment and religious rites performed with the patients and the families under the curanderas' leadership.

Diseases were understood to come from several sources. Some illnesses were the result of an imbalance in God's natural order caused by a careless accident or misuse of the body, some illnesses were thought to come from various kinds of bewitchments arising from purposeful evil on someone's part, some were thought to come from the evil eye, a force projected unknowingly by a person onto an envied object or person, and some illnesses were thought to be God's punishment for sin.

Various treatments were given, such as herbal teas, massage, poultices, and different kinds of cleansings. These treatments were accompanied by prayers and appeals to saints and attempts to set right again causes of imbalances or sources of bewitchments.

Three terms are used frequently when speaking of Hispanic folk curers. These terms are: curandera (curandero), *médica* (*medico*), and *partera*. In an attempt to differentiate between these terms, I interviewed five older residents coming from the villages of Trujillo, San Ignacio, and Sabinoso, and the cities of Santa Fe and Las Vegas. All five mentioned that the vast majority of the healers they had known were female. In addition, they stated that partera simply means midwife. A partera may be a médica or curandera, but not necessarily. The people also stated that a curandera relies more on magic and often deals with bewitchments as well as healing in general. Jesusita Aragón pointed out that today many young people considered curanderas to be old-fashioned and said, "Most of the kids now don't believe in curanderas, but years ago everybody did."

All the residents had heard the term médica used throughout their lives. The term implies some sort of advanced healing knowledge and extensive use of herbs or other techniques for healing. Many médicas were also parteras, but not necessarily. Jesusita Aragón, a partera, is also sometimes referred to as médica, while Julianita Baca had a wide reputation as a médica but did very little midwifery.[12]

Nevertheless, there were similarities among all of these healers, the curanderas, the médicas, and the parteras. They stressed the importance of harmony during pregnancy and the birth process. In addition, they were looked up to by the mothers and often turned to for advice and help with the many problems involved in child rearing and in general living. Many of these midwives and healers took an interest in the children they had delivered for the rest of the children's lives. Thus, the female healers were counselors and advice givers for the community, as well as medical practitioners and religious leaders, and they represented a centuries-old tradition of female medical care.

The Anglo medical system, introduced to these villages during the twentieth century, also had a high proportion of female medical care givers. A number of the early physicians in the area were female and when public health programs were brought to the county in the early 1930s most of those workers were women. They included nurses, nurse-midwives, and physicians.[13]

Today the medical system of the county closely approximates that of the rest of the nation and of the many midwives who used to practice in the area, only Jesusita remains. Yet, in many ways, Jesusita still maintains the tradition of the earlier lay midwives. Her medical services have a religious dimension in the prayers connected with births, her appeals to saints, and her understanding of midwifery as a God-given gift. As with the earlier parteras, she has taken a long term interest in the children she has delivered, and she uses herbs, teas, and massage in various treatments. In addition, she serves as a general counselor and source of referrals for the people in her community.[14] But to these traditions have been added modern medical hygiene, prenatal care and screening, and emergency backup.

Jesusita is the last of the traditional midwives to be licensed to practice in this part of New Mexico, and when she no longer is present, a particular tradition of female healing will have vanished. Yet, for the time being, many of the strengths and practices of the traditional female healers have stayed with the community, and the spirit of the healers continues.

Soon after I began work in New Mexico in early 1975 I was told about Jesusita by several friends who had babies with her. One commented that somebody should write Jesusita's life story. I was immediately interested and asked to be introduced to her. My friend and I walked the few blocks down a gravel road from the plaza to her aqua blue house that was set back from the road. We rang the doorbell, and Jesusita came to the door. She was a short, stocky woman with curled, closely cut brown and white hair. She had on sturdy shoes, a work dress, and one of the full sized aprons I came to associate with her. She hugged my friend and greeted me warmly and asked us to come and sit in her small, main room.

Jesusita was anxious to share her story with someone, and we eventually met together a number of times. The story is done in her words, the words of someone struggling to put the complexities and subtle memories of a full life in terms that can be understood by someone who speaks another language and comes from a different culture. I have not "corrected" her English, feeling her expressions have a special strength and reveal the uniqueness of people living in a bilingual culture. We tape recorded our many conversations and from the tapes I have organized the story of her life and work. These written words, however, can not convey the many visual nuances and details of sound and touch that were part of our relationship. As a consequence, I have recorded some details seen through my perspective that can help to portray her story.

I have many memories of Jesusita, but one of the clearest is of the lines and wrinkles of her body, especially of her hands and face. I also remember her touch, the touch of her arms as she embraced me, the memory of her hands stroking mine, holding them in times of greeting and parting, and touching them for reassurance or emphasis.

I also remember how she used her hands and arms to describe her midwife techniques: how to rub the uterus after birth, how and where to cut the cord, how to stroke a woman's back during hard labor, how to use fingers to massage the perineum during delivery, and how to ease out and support the breech birth. She also used her hands to illustrate many details of her past, the height of the grass outside her home as a child, the grass on land now nearly turned to desert, or the gestures of dances and games she and her friends played as children.

One of my most vivid visual recollections of Jesusita is her movement, her slow, expressive movements as she communicated to the outpatients and grandchildren she cared for, as she welcomed and arranged the seating for her patients and guests, as she made *tortillas*, scrubbed floors on her hands and knees, as she ran her wringer washer, and as she hung up the clothes of her grandchildren and outpatients. Finally, I especially remember the movements and touches involved in labor, birth, and the care of the newborn.

I picture her arranging her things for examination and birth, smoothing her bed, also used as a couch, and spreading out photos of her grandchildren and the babies she has delivered. I also picture her slowly stroking the arms of the rocking chair as she rocked back and forth and talked to me of her past and present life and troubles.

While we worked on the tapes Jesusita would answer the phone or door as many as eight times an hour. The interruptions came from many sources; some were her friends, from both out of town and in Las Vegas, who had come to share news or to ask for help with their troubles or to bring her herbs to use in her healings. She also had patients arrive at her door, women who were pregnant and needing help with deliveries or people coming for other reasons, asking her advice about going to a doctor, or seeking an herb or treatment for a wound or fever.

While meeting all these needs Jesusita maintained a host-like concern for all the people involved—for those in her bedroom–sitting room, for those attending another's birth, for those waiting to be checked themselves, and for those who had just come, like myself, to visit and share in her life. In addition, she frequently communicated by telephone with the extensions of her world, the state licensing people, the public health people, and the other local medical people.

At the same time Jesusita had a continual verbal and nonverbal relationship with her grandchildren and their friends as they came and went in her house, intertwining their lives with hers on a moment-by-moment basis. She was able to speak to me of times in the far past while she was simultaneously aware of the locations and activities of each of the mental hospital outpatients who boarded with her.

Yet, through all of this, she maintained extreme cleanliness and efficiency in her small home, the home that housed eight in addition to her patients. It was an area in which she maintained forceful control; almost no events occurred without her knowledge and rarely without her consent.

The space that she lived and worked in was deceptively small. The fifteen-foot-square, aqua colored main room served as both a combination bedroom for Jesusita herself and her eighteen-year-old granddaughter Martha and as a living room and waiting room for her patients. It held the double bed she and her granddaughter had shared since

Martha's young childhood. The rest of the furniture consisted of Jesusita's rocking chair and two small chairs that were used for guests. There were frequently a number of people in the room, and on those occasions some sat on the bed. In addition, the room contained her dresser with a surface filled with images and statues of saints and photos of relatives and friends. These had been placed carefully on hand worked doilies, were immaculately dusted, and had been in much the same position for the last ten years.

The room also included another wooden chest of drawers in which she kept her medical records and blank certificates. In the bottom drawer she kept plastic zippered folders containing information concerning her deliveries. She was especially proud of the books people had given her that displayed photographs of her deliveries and pictures of the children as they grew.

A small heater and a multitude of religious drawings and art were also in the room. There was a statue and painting of *San Antonio* and other paintings of *San Martín de Porres, San Martín Caballero, Nuestra Señora de Guadalupe, Santo Niño de Atocha,* and *San Ramón Nanato.* A carefully framed photograph of her mother and father taken shortly after their wedding was on one wall and a similarly framed photograph of President Kennedy was on another. Several crucifixes were also hanging in the room, and one of the chests proudly displayed a photo framed with patriotic emblems of her son in his army uniform.

The rest of the house similarly mirrored Jesusita's personality. In the three years I knew her I never saw a layer of dust or anything out of place. She cleaned and arranged constantly as she also did her midwife work and prepared food for the many residents of her home. I was often greeted at her main door by a combination smell of food cooking and strong, ammonia cleaner.

Next to the main room of her home was the delivery and examination room. It included a high, single bed with a firm mattress that was used for deliveries. Her granddaughter Martha once told me that when she was a young child and sleeping in the double bed in the adjoining room, she was often awakened during the night by the sounds of women giving birth. "I didn't like it," she said, "and would put the pillow over my head so I couldn't hear it and could go back to sleep." Then she smiled and continued, "Now I never hear it and sleep right through the whole thing."

Several chairs were also in the delivery room including one toward the end of the bed in which Jesusita sat while watching the course of the delivery. A suitcase containing the delivery materials was also stored there. It held a pan for the placenta, sterile string for the cord, scissors, a rubber suction bulb, and other materials. The room also had a bassinet and a scale to weigh the baby. The mothers were requested to bring other materials to the birth, including sterile sheets padded with newspaper and plastic, sterile cloth, cotton, and olive oil.

During a delivery, Jesusita arranged all of these materials in careful order so each could be reached immediately. Following the birth she would move with the baby to the kitchen and care for it there.

The delivery room also had a number of religious items on the walls, including a crucifix and paintings of *Domingo de Ramas, San Luis,* and San Antonio. A painting of Nuestra Señora de Guadalupe hung above the bed and was positioned so the mother in labor could fix her eyes on it. The painting of San Luis had belonged to her great grandmother.

In addition, the small house included an entrance hall, a bath and laundry room, a kitchen, and a back wing leading from the delivery room. She had built the wing and used it originally as a four patient maternity ward. But when she no longer had as many deliveries, she began to use the wing to house four male outpatients from the state mental hospital. Thus, her meager income was supplemented by state payments for her care of these men. As a consequence, all her projects, her family, her home, her maternity work, and the outpatients she cared for, were housed together.

Her forty-six-year-old son, Ernesto, had built his small house immediately in front of hers and had added a room that joined the two houses for his son, Steve. Steve, aged fifteen, was the youngest member of her household.

One other community besides Las Vegas had special importance in the story of Jesusita's life, that is the village of Trujillo, near which she lived as a child and young adult, and
the ranch where she grew up. On a hot August day, her
granddaughter Martha and I set out to visit the area where
so many events in Jesusita's life history had occurred.
Trujillo is located on the plains about forty-two miles directly east of Las Vegas. We drove east for about an hour on
a fairly straight highway through a desolate and largely
abandoned area. What had formerly been the llanos, plains
of high grass, had changed drastically through the droughts
of the last forty years. The grasses found there now are
scraggly and separated into strawlike clumps, not over eight
inches high. Cactus and sage brush also grow in with the
sparse grass.

Occasional canyons divide up the rust and beige dirt and
cut with meandering lines into the relatively flat plains.
Scrub oak, juniper, and piñon trees grow in the canyons and
add deep greens to the rust and tan of the earth. Above it all
is the ever present blue sky stretching the vast distances to
the horizon.

A number of sparrows were disturbed as we traveled
down the highway. They flew up quickly as we approached
and settled back down to their normally still road. We saw
ravens scavenging the dry land and an occasional hawk soar-
ing out over the immense span.

These birds were almost the only sign of life except for
scattered old stone and adobe homes. Most of the homes
looked totally abandoned, but some still showed signs of
life. We stopped at one of the homes and visited with Jesusita's half brother's wife. Martha talked with her in Spanish,
asking her about her health and her recent operation while
the woman served us sandwiches and water. She then described a fork in the road at which we should turn left in
order not to miss Trujillo. As we drove on we also passed a
number of old windmills. Most of the windmills were too
broken to move but some creaked slowly around in the
wind.

We eventually reached Trujillo itself which consisted of a
small clump of deteriorating buildings. Three men sat in

the shade of one of the buildings. One of the men came over, and Martha told him why we had come and what we were looking for. He called to another, an older man, Pedro Baca, who had known Jesusita when they were young. The older man came out of the shade into the white sun and pointed to the rutted, dirt road we should take to the site of the ranch.

We drove on for several miles and came to an old windmill whose blades had broken and were lying scattered on the ground. This was the Aragón windmill that Jesusita had described to me with such love and pride. I looked at its broken base and the pieces lying around it and remembered that this windmill had given the whole family water, water that for years had been carried in buckets from the spring one and one-half miles away. I thought of the mass that had been held beneath the windmill to celebrate its presence and how priests had come from Las Vegas to perform the rite. It had begun to rain during the mass, but the service went on, and the family had been filled with happiness.

We went to the small house beyond and visited briefly with elderly Gregorio and Eloisa Parson. They spoke gently about the years when Jesusita had lived near them, remembering when Dolores, Ernesto, and Ben were children and how Gregorio had taught Ernesto how to play the guitar. They showed us the house of Jesusita's married sister, Soledad, the building which Jesusita had described as a grand white house with flowers planted around it. The house was now used to store hay, and when we walked into its coolness out of the hot sun, a barn swallow flew from its nest in the eaves and out through the broken door. I bent down and picked up the remains of a child's shoe, the only remnant of the three sisters' families that had lived so close to each other.

We finally found what was left of Jesusita's home, the home she had built by herself when she was sent out from her family's house because of her two unmarried pregnancies. Only a twenty-foot square of medium-sized rocks remained; the wood she had cut and formed had been sold long ago. Several piñon had grown up by the house since Jesusita and her children had left, and we stood quietly for a minute and listened to the ever present wind blowing through the trees. Even the stones were gone from the site of Jesusita's sister Ramona's house. Like Jesusita, Ramona too had moved out of her family's house following an unmarried pregnancy. The two sisters had lived near to each other for six years, raising their children alone, until Ramona died and Jesusita took Ramona's young son, Ben, into her home.

Later we stopped at Ramona's grave. Martha identified it by a bouquet of plastic flowers Jesusita had placed there years before. The wooden cross was broken, one side was missing, and an ant hill had developed on the dry, rocky earth of the grave. Martha straightened the remaining piece of cross, pushed away the ant hill with her shoe and a stick, and recentered the pink plastic flowers.

We went further on down the incredibly bumpy road until the road simply stopped. We had reached a group of abandoned buildings, the buildings in which Jesusita's aunts and uncles had lived and worked. There were no sounds anywhere except for the constant wind and the occasional calls of birds. We suddenly heard the startled scurry of a small animal, but then it was silent again.

We hiked down into the canyon, knowing this was part of the ranch in which Jesusita had herded sheep and goats as a child. The wind blew harder here through the more numerous cedar, juniper, and piñon, and the large rocks and boulders presented a more familiar mountain landscape. We remembered Jesusita's warning about rattlesnakes and watched where we walked and listened carefully as we moved. The canyon sides were more moist than above, and the grass and bushes were higher.

On the way back through Trujillo we located the church which had been newly built when Jesusita lived in the area. It too had fallen into disarray. We also located the school building that had been the site of many of the dances that Jesusita had enjoyed so deeply and the larger cemetery containing the graves of relatives and friends.

I returned to Trujillo nearly a year later. Jesusita's son, Ernesto, accompanied me to help me find the location of her grandparents' home, the home in which her son and daughter had been born.

It was early summer, and for several weeks we had been having afternoon thundershowers; consequently, the land was much greener and more alive than the August before. The small clumps of grama grass and rabbit brush were green, and red, yellow, and purple wildflowers were in bloom. Even the cactus, yucca, and thistle contributed to the color. The birds seemed as alive as the flowers, and we heard meadowlarks sing and saw hawks and crow soar above.

We hiked a mile or so down into the canyon along a washed out rock path that had once been the road. The canyon was beautiful, the sky and air clear, and we could see many miles to the blue mountains on the horizon.

We eventually came to the remains of the buildings. Jesusita's grandparents' home was built of stone. Stone walls, wood window frames, and a door frame were all that remained of the main section of the house. Stones scattered in a rough rectangle and a few weathered boards outlined a wooden addition, and one corner of a fence and two horseshoes gave evidence of the corral.

I went inside the stone house, and through the windows I could see the remains of a neighbor's wooden home. No people came to these homes now except Jesusita's brother who occasionally rides down on horseback. We took the horseshoes with us as we left, climbed back up the walls of the canyon, and drove back to town.

I have one memory that I connect vividly with these visits. The memory is of Jesusita telling me that when she was a young woman the grass had grown "this high" around the little home she built for herself and her children. As she spoke she indicated a height of about two-and-one-half feet from the floor. While she was speaking I pictured the square of rocks and near desert landscape there now. I also knew from records and stories that large crops were grown on the land that is so arid today. These vivid contrasts have stayed in my memory, along with the stories of those people who lived out their lives in that vast place.

The following, then, is the story of Jesusita Aragón. The story is told in her own words and contains glimpses into the lives of many others. Many of the names have been changed to protect people's privacy, but the facts of their hard, and useful, lives remain the same.

Childhood in Trujillo

WE LIVED IN TRUJILLO when I was little, but when they start to build the lake, the Storrie Lake by Las Vegas, my daddy came back to Las Vegas and asked for work, for work building the dam 'cause we needed the money. So we moved back here to Upper Town in Las Vegas for awhile.

My mother got pregnant again, her eighth baby. All girls. Eight girls, trying to have a boy. Only three girls lived. I was the first that lived. Then my two little sisters. There was alot of death then 'cause they don't have any doctors here. Just do something that you think is good for it, to try and cure that people. My five sisters died when they were little. Between four, two, and one. From different kinds of sickness. There was much death and much sorrow.

Then in 1918, when I was ten, the bad flu came. A lot of people die on that time. 1918. A lot of people die. One of my uncles. And little ones too, my relatives' little ones. But I didn't get it, and I help take care of everybody. They ask for some water, something to eat, but they never touch it. They couldn't.

My mother was pregnant when she got sick. And she last three days, and she couldn't talk no more. She start with a pain on her back, and it come through her chest so she couldn't talk. She writes to my grandmother when she wants something. And her tears run. I cry and she cries. I was scared, and I stayed with her.

She was about seven months with the baby. The doctor took care of her and said it was better for her to have the baby than to die with the baby in because she was not going to last too long. And the doctor gave her something to make her have the baby. She could still talk a little then, and she knew she was to have the baby, so she said, "Jesusita, call your aunt, tell her that I have my baby," 'cause my grandmother was at the ranch. But that day my grandmother come. My grandmother delivered it by herself; nobody was with her, just the neighbors, right here in Upper Town. It was another girl, the last one. I heard that baby cry. The baby girl last about an hour, I think, and then she die. I think my mother didn't feel anything; she was so sick. And in a few days my mother die. She was thirty-four.

I was ten years old when my mother died, and the other sister was five, and the little one, the little sister, was three years old. We cried and cried and were sad, but my grandmother and aunts were with us.

We couldn't go to the funeral because it was a big storm, a snow in March. We felt such sorrow because we couldn't go, and our mother was gone. I slept with my sisters and helped them when they missed our mother. I remember I give them a bath and comb their hairs. Yes, I cleaned my sisters when our mother died. And my daddy missed her so; he felt much sadness for our mother.

My mama and daddy had met right here in Las Vegas. My daddy was nineteen when he met my mother at a dance, and they got married when they were twenty-one. They are twenty-one in the picture I have of them, the picture on my wall. Everybody tell me that she looked so pretty when she was a bride.

They got married right there near the drive-in, right there where those pictures are on the roof, the A and W. There was a church there years ago, a small church. I used to see the church and remember. I don't forget; I don't forget anything. Now the church is gone, and there is the A and W, but I remember.

I was born here on a hill by the Storrie Lake, and they baptized me at Sapello. I was my mother's third baby, her third girl. The others die.

My mother was the only sister in her family, and they never forget her. They used to call her Tonia. Her name was Antonia, and we call her Tonita. Mama Tonita. After I was born, when I was three, my family can't make their living with the farm anymore. They have to move because they don't have a ranch here. They have too many goats, too many sheep, and they didn't have enough place to keep it. They went to the courthouse and see what place is free. I think they homesteaded; maybe that's what it was called. The land wasn't used by anybody. They were the first people there. It was by a village called Trujillo.

I don't remember anything about when we moved; I was three years old. But I know we moved in the summer in three wagons, from here to there, and we lived in a tent until they make their homes. We lived together, my two uncles, my aunt, my grandfather, my grandmother, my father, my mother, my sisters, and me. And little by little, they fix their own homes out of wood cut from trees and mud to use to patch it. Yes, they make a little village, and later they build with stone. There was a spring in the canyon, about a mile and a half from our house. We carry the water up in buckets back then and take the sheep and the goats to the spring.

We had all lived together in Trujillo before my daddy came back to work at Storrie Lake and before my mama died. I remember too much. I never forget my parents, never. There is nothing in the world like your mother. That's your best friend. I never forget her or forget how she looks or how she holds me. If I'd had my mother I would never have been put out of the house later. Never. She would have been good to me.

After my mother die, we go back to the ranch in Trujillo, and my grandmother takes care of us. My daddy came too. We were all together. With my grandfather, I don't know how to tell you, because he spoiled me. That's why they called me Tita, because my grandfather called me Tita. He sits me on his arms, and he say, "My dear Tita, I love you, Tita."

You know how my daddy used to call me? *Amigo.* Because when my mother was pregnant he was thinking that I'm going to be a boy. So that's why he called me amigo. "*Mi amigo*, mi amigo," always, "mi amigo." It made me feel good, and I wish I was a boy, but I wasn't.

But when people ask my daddy, "How do you feel with too many girls," he said, "I feel OK. I feel OK. I don't change one of my girls for two boys." But I was raised out like a man, like a boy. I don't know why. Maybe because my daddy don't have any other boys, not till I was eighteen. Maybe that's why I was raised out like a boy. They never whip me. No, never. Other kids got whipped. They used to whip their kids years ago, but they never whip me, nobody. I was lucky that way, I know. Because when I see my aunts or my uncles whipping their kids, oh, I cry for them. I cry for them because they never do that with me. Neither my uncles. When something's wrong, they talk to me. Just talk to me and tell me, "Don't do that again. We don't want to whip you; we like you too much." That's what they told me; I guess because I'm the oldest in the house.

Also, they just look at us with their eyes. A special way. You know, so nobody know but you. Now, if you make them eyes at kids, they say, "Why do you make me that." It is so, but then we obey.

They are all gone now. I have every kinds of sadness. A lot of death. My father, my grandparents, my aunts and uncles, everybody. They're all gone. Only one old uncle is left. Isidro Gallegos. He's in his eighties. When I was a little girl he sits me on his shoulder and walks with me to see the sheeps, the cows, and everything on the ranch. So I love him. He's the only one left; that's all I have now.

Oh, the ranch was beautiful then. We had so much. The grass grows high from the ground. Green and pretty. We had birds; we had mockingbirds and doves and eagles and owls and crows. And the sky always so blue.

We had plenty of deer. They get near the house and drink water and eat some salt where the sheeps and goats eat the salt. They get near but aren't scared because we never hurt them. Big and small. I know them as soon as they're born. Little deer with three rows of white spots on their backs. I know each of them.

Oh, I liked to work outside then. I like the sun, the wind, and everything. Rain. I used to hope for the rain. That's a good hope, the rain, and I like it.

But when it doesn't rain we never have water. Later they dig a well, but before they dig that well, we used to bring the water from the spring, a mile and a half far. Oh, it was sweet and good water. We're glad to have it, but you can't get it in a wagon or nothing, you have to go walking for it. And for the animals we have to go real far to a canyon. One day after another we go on horses to water the sheep. You take all day long to water the goats and the sheeps. They drink water, and they turn to another way. They learn how to come back, but we have to watch them.

We had fields then. We got big fields with beans, corn, peas, cane, wheat, oh, everything. We make a big garden too, with beets, onions, peanuts, and cucumbers, with everything in the garden. Chili, green chili; we make our living pretty good.

We had sheeps and goats, two thousand sheeps and five hundred goats. And cows and hogs. We didn't have to buy anything, not even lard, and they made our syrup out of cane. Just coffee, sugar, that's all we have to buy.

The corn, when it grows, if you get in that field on horseback you can't see the men on it. They were tall, tall canes and crops, and the ear corn is the big size. We used to can everything, so in winter we don't have to buy anything.

And we have pigs, sheep, goats, cattle. And they used to kill one of each one so we make the lard. We dry the meat and make some *chicharrones*, and we make our butter there. Cream, we didn't have to buy it, just put your spoon in there and get your cream or butter, whatever you want. We have everything then, everything.

Yes, my daddy used to have a big, big crops. And everybody, because the road was near the fence, everybody took some peas, watermelons, or corn, whatever they want to from my daddy's field. He doesn't care. No, he was a good man. "If I have, everybody have." That's the way he said.

Some times are hard, though. Sometimes the little calves or lambs or little goats were dying and, well, it's a bad year for those. That's when my grandfather used to say, "*Dios da y Dios quita.* The Lord gives and the Lord takes away. Don't worry," he says. "Dios da y Dios quita." Those were hard years, but mostly there were good.

Long ago children worked with adults. That way everybody learns how to work. And we all work together picking some beans or something. My father, grandparents, aunts, uncles, and cousins. We help each other.

And we eat together sometimes. My grandmother has a long table and a big kitchen, and everybody sits around that table. The big first, and then the small ones. And somebody else was there to serve them and to take care of the kids.

The old ones are gone now, and some of the little ones live in California, Colorado, and Texas. And when they come to visit here, everybody come and see me. Because they treat me like a grandma. Everybody comes, "Hello Tita; hello little Tita." They hug me and give me a kiss, and everybody treats me good. And I like them like they were my sons and daughters. Since they were babies, I know them.

It was good to eat together, very good. But I don't like to cook, not too much. I pay my sisters, and they have to cook. I pay them to cook for me, and I work outside. Well, I don't like cooking; I have to do it anyway, but I don't like it.

We had two big families in Trujillo. We are the Aragóns and the other is the Gallegos. Everybody there have his own place to plant and to have their own animals. They make fences and separate the places. Sometimes the animals get over the fences, but we fix the fence and put them back. And nobody fight. We get along pretty good with everybody. Everybody goes to the same church and the same school.

Oh, my grandfather had a big place, and it was my grandfather's spring. But when he die everybody takes his part. My daddy and all the others. But now even the windmill doesn't work. It broke, and nobody cares for it. Now there are just a few left. Where we used to live, so many of us, there is just one. He buys my daddy's ranch and my uncles' and his father-in-law's. He buys everything. Now there's just a few, but then there were so many.

Yes, I work outside like a man back then; I was raised out like a boy. Sometimes I think it would be better to be a boy. It's easy to be raised for a boy. You can go and work wherever you want. And for a girl is different. You can go somewhere else and work, but it's different to get along. People are stricter with a girl. Can't try as many things if a girl. But I do many things like a boy.

But I wear my hair like a girl back then, long and in braids, two braids. And my grandmother has long, long hair, almost to her heels. Her head was so heavy we have to help her wash it in a tub, and then she didn't comb it till it was dry. Yes, she had good black hair, my grandmother did.

My grandmother also used long skirts everywhere. And we used to wear a long skirt when we go to the dances or masses. But I wear jeans to ride and take care of the sheeps. And I wear jeans when I went on horses to deliver babies. Because I don't sit on horses like my grandmother sits. No. She sits across the saddle, sideways, but she didn't fall down. She can run and do how she wants on horseback, and she didn't fall. Every woman used to ride like her. But they didn't teach me to ride that way.

They teach me to ride like a boy. And when we have big *fiestas* over there, and I have to take care of the sheeps and everybody was at the fiesta, I have to come by myself on horseback, like a boy. Not like a girl, like a boy. And nobody bothers me, no. Everybody likes me.

I went all day on my horse with my dogs to watch the sheep. I move them around and don't let them go apart, they have to be together all the time. It's not hard to watch the sheep when you're used to take care of them. And I sing and play the harmonica while I watch the sheep. I sing lots of tunes, and I always have my harmonica here in my pocket in my shirt. Always. I teach myself to play it.

We have to go far to the canyon to water the sheep and goats. But I ride my horse, and he picks his way over the rocks and grass and cactus down in the canyon. One day after another I go to water the sheep.

When they were having their babies, the lambs and goats, it's hard to take the mothers down there to water them 'cause the babies stay up here. Little lambs and little goats crying and crying and running away. They don't want to stay here. They just get all together and cry, cry, and cry until the mothers come up from the spring. We have to watch the little ones so they don't scatter all over. It is a lot of work to do. And we do it.

When it rained and I was out far with the sheeps I have to stay there, taking care of them. I get under a rock or under a good tree. Sometimes I'm scared. Real scared. I cry and pray and have my dogs, one on one side and the other on the other side. I cry for my mother. You know what I said? "Oh, dear mother. If I have you I wouldn't be here." She wouldn't make me work outside like that. I would be able to stay home, but the others don't care for me like my mother.

The sheep and goats go under trees when we have a big storm. And when we have a big hail sometimes it hurts them. Or kill them if it's a big one, and it hits them on the head. We used to lost too many sometimes. And when lightening kills one, and if there is a bunch of them, it kills all of them. And you can't eat the meat, it gets black. No, we never used it.

But I'm not too afraid then. I just pray, pray the Lord to take care of me. I'm not afraid now. No, I'm not too afraid of anything. I don't know why, but maybe because I was raised out like a man, like a boy. When I'm little I go out by myself, day or night. When we have something to do at night I wasn't scared. And I'm not scared now. If I hear something outside I'll go out and see what's the matter. What is making the noise or something. Sometimes the only sound is the trash cans. Nobody scares me. If a man comes here, and I don't know him, I'm not scared. My daddy teaches me to never get scared. That way they won't hurt you. But if you feel that you're afraid, they do it more and more to frighten you. But they can't frighten me so easy, no.

I tell my grandson, my granddaughter, "Don't be afraid of nobody. Nobody will hurt you." 'Cause I wasn't afraid.

If my daddy told me, "Jesusita, go and bring me this or that," whatever he needs. "Go out and see what's the matter with the chickens, they are crying. Maybe it's a coyote or another dog 'cause there are too many dogs that like to get the chickens," I wasn't afraid. I get the rifle, the .22, and I go out and see. They teach me how to shoot. I know how to manage the .30-30, the .22, or a pistol, the .38. But I never go hunting, we don't need the meat. I just shoot rattle-snakes.

I take care of the rattlesnakes when I'm out with the sheeps and goats. I watch for the snakes, and I kill the rat-tlesnakes with a .22. It's easier to kill them with a .22 than a rock. Sometimes I see a bunch of snakes together. I see them when they are breeding. They get round on each other, and they can bite you and eat you in a little while. 'Cause a lot of them get together. It is frightening because when they see you, they scatter, so you don't know where to run. Also, sometimes when they are alone I come close to step-ping on them, but they rattle and I run away. I had the chance, thanks to God.

They never hurt me, and they hurt nobody from the family. But sometimes they bite the animals, and some-times the animals die. We try to take care of them. We cut that part and squash it. We take care of our hand and wash the wounds with some herbs, and we put some salt in the wound. Sometimes the animals live through, but often they die.

When I'm just a little older I help to shear the sheep. We sharpen the scissors on a round grinder and bring the sheep into the corral. I put the sheep down with my knees and left hand and cut the wool with my right. Then we make a little bundle, every sheep that we shear. We make that wool into a bundle and tie it and put it in a sack.

We start early in the morning, and we quit when it's get-ting dark, 'cause we have too many sheeps. Sometimes it takes a week to do it, sometimes a little more if it rains, 'cause the wool has to be dry. I used to shear sixty or sixty-five in a day, and I have a cousin, José Gallegos, and he shears one hundred in a day.

After we're done we bring it into town in three or four wagons, and when my grandfather gets to town, to the ware-house, they give him a big cigar and light it for him 'cause he's rich. They make a contract with him and pay him for the wool.

No other girls know how to do it, but I know how to shear, and I work outdoors like a boy. I don't like indoor work, but I have to do it too. I have to help my grandmother with the house. I work outside all day, and then at night I do girls' work, the indoor work.

We get up about 4:00 in the morning, so we can do everything, and we go to bed as soon as we eat supper, and we sleep real swell 'cause we're so tired. After supper I like to sit on the floor with my back against the wall, so I can rest that way. I take my shoes off, wash my feet, and rest and rest.

Sometimes the cattles, sheep, and goats can't have their babies, and I have to help them. Often the young cattle, just two or three years old, have trouble with their first calf.

When I bring the sheep and goats to the ranch in the evening and I know some cattle is missing, I go where they eat or where they drink water.

When I find those cattle, and they're having trouble with the calves, I put a little rope around the nose and front hooves of the baby calf stuck in the mother, and I pull gently. I help pull that little calf out.

After I'm older sometimes the neighbors have trouble with their animals, and they come to ask me for help. One of my neighbors, he has too many problems with his goats and sheep. One goat is born with no front legs, and one set of twins are born dead and connected at the back. So I tell him how to change; to change the males with some other neighbor, so he can get good sheep and goats. I teach him how to breed.

I work hard, but I have fun too, long ago when I was a girl. I had good times with my animals. I had two dogs to help me with the sheeps. I get the little dogs before they open their eyes and get two goats, one for each dog, and I nurse those dogs from the goats. And that goat learns to like the little dog. When they start to suck, oh, the goats jumped and jumped because those dogs used to scratch the breast, but they get used to it. The dogs grow and take care of me and the sheeps. One of them, his name was Galafre. Galafre was the best bullfighter in Spain years ago, and my grandfather choose that name. And the other one was Spot. They helped me with the coyotes when I was out with the sheep.

I also had a pet goat when I was little that I raise.

Machivita, that's what I call her. When I was far, I call her, "Chivita, *vente*." That means "come here," and she cries and jumps and comes to me. She stands up and puts her hands up on my shoulders. Oh, I like her.

I also have a mare. *Tumbaga* was her name. Tumbaga was an old ring years ago, a real gold ring, and my horse was gold with a white spot on her forehead.

For fun I used to race on my horse with my uncle, Isidro Gallegos. He was ten years older than me and the one who teaches me how to ride. I usually win 'cause I'm lighter than him. I love riding fast on Tumbaga with the wind in my hair.

We had too many horses back then, and my uncle helps me break them. He would get on a horse and hold the other horse for me as I ride, and that's how we teach the horses.

I was happy back then on my horse or just climbing on the rocks in the canyon. I was just like a little goat, hopping from rock to rock, singing and whistling and making noise.

My grandma says, "Aren't you tired? Don't you get tired making all that noise?"

And I say, "No, I don't get tired. I am happy." And I don't get tired today, just my feet sometimes.

Oh, we had good times when I was little. I remember playing outside, playing in the water when the water was falling. I like to play outside without shoes; all of us like to play outside in the water when it is raining. I remember other times too, jumping rope and swinging. We put some swings on a tree, and we had dances under the trees. We all get together, neighbors and my cousins and my sisters, and I play the harmonica, and we dance. I know then how to call those square dances, but I forget now. And when we don't have a harmonica to play with our dances, we use a comb with a paper on the back to make music. We have a big, big tree, and it was clean where they dance all around. We have fun then. That's what I tell these kids now, that we learned how to play, how to read, how to talk on the hard way. Not like now. It's easy, everything is easy now.

About thirty of us play together then. Not every day, sometimes Sundays, sometimes a Saturday afternoon 'cause we were working all the time. We could just play a little while, then they call, "Come on and make dinner." Or wash the dishes, or sweep the floors, something. No, they don't let us play too long, just a little while, about an hour or two, but it was fun.

Also, I learn to dance, and I love to dance, then and now. They teach me in the house, my grandfather, my uncles, my daddy, everybody teach me how to dance. The first dance I went to when I was twelve years old. I remember it well, and I dance there with everybody. Gregario Parson and my uncles play the music. We had all kinds of tunes, all kinds. They used to play *cuadrillas*, like square dances, and waltz, polkas, everything over. We have guitar and violin. I especially like to waltz.

We have dances every fifteen or twenty days. That's all we have over there, dances and mass. The boys arrange the dances, because they want to see if their girl friends are there. They rent the hall and pay the music, and then they'd go everywhere saying, "Tonight we're going to have a dance." No radio, no thing then. So they went around the village, and the girls got excited.

But sometimes our family don't let us come. If you ask them, "Can you take us to the dance tonight, Grandma?"

"No, and don't tell me again, that's all."

So I cry all night under my blankets. Because I love dances. So, we don't have to ask again, just once, and if they say yes, that's yes.

But if they say once, "No and that's it; don't ask me anymore," then I would cry.

My sisters, they said, "You're crazy." Yes, I was crazy, that's right, 'cause I love dances.

When we were little they used to tell us stories, and I remember too many things that my grandmother and my grandfather used to talk with me. They used to talk that way to the kids when they get together, and we believe on everything. And now they don't believe, no. If you tell kids a story, they say, "Oh, I already know it." That's sad, 'cause it's fun to tell stories.

They told us stories about Cinderella and witches. They told us that years ago when a *bruja*, a witch, wants to go outside and visit all the villages, it was a big ball of fire. And when I was little I saw too many things like that right there on the ranch, but I wasn't afraid 'cause they used to talk with me about those things. Just knowing about the stories made me feel safe.

My daddy used to tell us stories about Vicente Silva and his gang of forty thieves. Silva killed lots of people and his wife too because he wants to go with another woman. My daddy knew those thieves; my daddy knew everybody, but they didn't hurt him. They like him a lot when my daddy was a boy.

They told us stories from *La Historia Sagrada*, like the New Testament. My father learned stories by memory, but he can't read English, just Spanish. We all get together, and they tell the stories to us. We sit together in the evening. It was good feelings. Oh, I know too many things, but it's hard to remember. But I remember too many things they used to tell me.

I remember other things like coming to Las Vegas with my grandfather. I come with my grandfather every year when they bring the wool to sell, or they sell the little goats, and later, when I am older, I drive one wagon with the sacks of wool. My grandmother and grandfather come in the buggy then, and my daddy and uncle drive two other wagons filled with wool.

And we come when they have rodeos for the Fourth of July, the fiesta time. We start from Trujillo at 3:00 in the morning on a wagon, and we get here about 11:00 and stay here two or three days. Oh, we had a good time. They have everything in the rodeo, roping, bulldogging, riding bronco bulls, everything. They have stands everywhere to sell too many things, and they have a big parade. It was fun and so pretty. Now they don't have anything, just a little parade, no rodeos, no nothing.

Later, when I am older, we have a 4-H Club, and the people from the club take things we make to the state fair. I made it with my hand, no machine. I used to sew, very, very thin, and when somebody's getting married there, they bring me their outfit so I fix it, with my hand. I sew for too many people. We got together to can for the fair and in the schoolhouse to sew, crochet, embroider. We had good times together, and we win prizes.

We had many special things back then. We had a saint we believed on. *Santo Niño de Atocha* is our saint. We all believe on him because, you know, when the oldest one believe on this saint the youngest ones learn to believe on it too. The family fix a little throne outside for the Three, and they put that Santo Niño there. The Santo Niño is a child and sits on a chair. He helps us with hard times. In the summertime we pray to him and ask him to watch the fields, to give us a good crop and help us with the rain. And he did; he help everybody. And we tell him, "Don't send no hail." Sometimes we have hail, but the plants come out again. We say the rosary there, in the morning and at night.

But nobody believes on these things now, no. These kids don't believe it. They say, "That's an old-fashioned." You know, that's what they say. I feel mad with them. My grandchildren don't say that, but other kids, lots do.

A neighbor of mine was here a few days ago. They still live out by Trujillo. She was saying she remembers when we got together and pray and have faith, and she say that nobody has faith now. She says that's why we don't have any rain, and I think that's right. They don't care too much; they don't care. Years ago they used to make masses under a tree or under a well, something like that. We put an altar and then we have the mass there. It was pretty, and everybody come to that, everybody, walking or horseback or wagons or cars, different ways. Sometimes it starts raining when we were there, and we never quit, we stay there. The priest never quits either. It felt good to have the rain come. We're glad to have that rain. Sometimes we have rain everyday. It doesn't rain now, though. They don't do any farming neither. Nobody. They can't; there is no rain.

For too many years back then we carry water from the spring in buckets. Then when I was grown, we dig a well and build a windmill. We promise to our Lord, if he give us some water, 'cause we are tired to bring water so far, we would make our Lord a mass there, at the windmill. And he did, we got water. So we ask the priest to go and give us a mass at our windmill, and a lot of people went there. We make a little altar under the mill.

And the rain came when we were there. Nobody leave,

we stay there, and the rain came and came. We had a lot of rain that day, and nobody went home, they stay until the father finish with the mass.

I was religious then, very religious. I don't have a chance to go to mass now, but I don't forget my prayers, oh no. I used to pray the stations and the rosaries. I know how to pray very well, and I can sing. I know too many *himnos*. My grandmother taught me all those things.

Yes, we were thankful to our Lord for our windmill back then, but now it's broken. It's all down, and nobody fixes it. Nobody takes care of those things. Our good windmill.

We have pretty occasions back then, pretty occasions and too many things, for Christmas, New Year's, *Corpus Christi*, and for the San Ysidro. On May 15 we celebrate the San Ysidro. Everybody gets together and three or four priests, they celebrate that day, the 15 of May. San Ysidro is our saint of the fields. He has a team of ox and a wooden plow, and we love him. We have a big *santo* of San Ysidro inside the church, about three or four feet high, and a small one that we carry with the ox in the procession.

In May, the first days of May, everybody comes together and cleans the church and gets ready for the *función*. We fix around the church with pines and wild flowers. We have four *mayordomos*. They take care of the church and clean the church and everything inside and outside during the year, and on the 15 of May they change. These ones name another ones so they have to take care of the church the next year. I am one a year when I was older, me and my son Ernesto.

And then on May 15 we have a big mass first and then a *procesión*. The priests go first, and then the choir, the choir goes behind them. Then the mayordomos carry the saint, *San Ysidro*, and the little *bueys*, the little ox. Then the other people walk, singing and praying, and we go round the church a few times. There is violins and guitars, and the bells are ringing, and we are singing and praying as we go around the church.

Then afterwards we have dinner all together, a big, big dinner. Sometimes we have a barbeque, and I am one of the cooks and Carolina Madrid, the best cook in all Trujillo. She was my father's sister-in-law. I can cook, but not like her, and then after the dinner we have a big dance. The dance is at night, but sometimes at daytime we dance too. But we are too busy, mostly, cooking and doing dishes to dance till night. Wow, that's a good day we had. We have another special time on our Corpus Christi. We have the little girls who take their first communion all dressed in white with veils. We teach them to sing and pray and go in the procesión. They're our *niñas de Maria*, and they lead us on the day. We make a pretty altar outside with saints and flowers and branches of trees. The priest goes in front and leads us around and around the church. Then the girls come singing and throwing flowers and our San Ysidro and the people in the back. We stop at the altar each time around, and the priest says prayers and sings, and then we go into the church and have high mass.

Oh, it is pretty too, and the girls are so proud. When I'm older I teach them how to sing, and then I help with the big dinner after.

Those are good memories, good memories, but they won't come back. No, they never come back. Now it's not the same. The priest still goes to give mass, but every two or three months. They still go some, but it's not the same.

My father married again after my mother died. I like my stepmother OK, but sometimes she's hard on me. I didn't care, though, because I was with my grandmother. When my stepmother starts to nag, nag, nag, I went out of her house and to my grandma's house. My grandmother and my grandfather raised me. My father and stepmother had more children. I have six half sisters and two half brothers. My first brother was born when I was eighteen, and I help raise them all, but three of them died.

When I'm seventeen my daddy gets Matias. Matias was seven years old when he comes with my daddy. His father was my daddy's first cousin, and his mother was my god mother. Matias's daddy dies, and his mother has eight kids to feed on just $3.00 a week. She makes it cleaning houses, ironing clothes, and washing clothes for other people, and eight kids she tries to feed.

So when my daddy comes to town, to get our food and everything, Matias says, "I'm going with you." And he was a good boy. My father didn't have to bother with him 'cause Daddy'd say, "We're going to do this today," and Matias would do it. I don't like to go anywhere in those years. I was always like that back then. Sometimes when my daddy and his wife go to see her daddy's in La Centa, sometimes I feel like going with them to talk with her sisters. You see, there were twelve in her family.

My daddy and stepmother go in the wagon, and I like to go on horseback. But when I get to the hill where I can stretch up on my horse and see my grandparents' house I start to cry and say, "Daddy, I don't want to go with you. My grandfather and grandmother might get sick, and I wouldn't be here with them."

So, he says, "OK, that's OK if you don't want to go. You can stay with them."

And I don't go to visit people with them. Just if I go the same day and back. I'm supposed to be there with my people, there with the ones I love.

I started to school when I was six, before my mother died. We have seats for two in the school, and the kids are six to sixteen years old. We had maybe forty kids and two teachers. They teach just in Spanish, and the older kids help the younger kids. The kids never fight with me, never, and I never fight with nobody. I don't like to fight.

When I'm eleven, I start to learn English. I learn English by reading. My uncle Steven had a book, Spanish and English. On one side was English and the other, the same page, Spanish. He reads it so I could hear, and I learned English that way.

Nobody in my house but me knows English, so, when Anglo people want to ask for a store or which way to go to find somebody else, nobody knows what they say, and they send for me where I was working. Now I speak an old-fashioned English like they speak years ago, a years ago language.

I finish school at eighth grade. I want to go to school more so much. I want to come over here to Las Vegas and finish, but, you know, they never like education, "No," they say,

"Oh, no, no. It's enough; you don't need anymore." So I quit, but I'm sad.

There are so many things to learn back then. So many things for the girls. The girls don't even know what it is when you have your period. They never let you know anything, and the girls get scared because they don't know anything. But I learn it from my aunts. My aunts tell me, and then I show my sisters. So when we have our period we already know, because of my aunts. I have two, Sophia and Petra. And I told my granddaughters, too, and when their mothers tell them something, they say, "Don't tell me anything. Tita show me."

Back then most girls don't know what's happening when they get married. They get scared. They don't want to lay down with him, oh no. They have to fight with her because they used to talk with me afterwards. "Oh," they say, "it's awful, it's awful." You get scared, and I don't blame them because they don't know anything. Sometimes they get pregnant, and they are ashamed to tell their mothers. Nobody knows anything, 'cause of the mothers. I don't know why the mothers are ashamed to tell them about it; I don't know.

But my grandmother used to tell me everything. She teach me everything, and I like to hear what is this or that and that and that. So I learn. I don't know why, but I always said that I'm going to be a midwife, and she used to tell me, "Yeah, you better be, because when I die you're going to be the one that takes care of everybody here at the ranch." And that was true.

Yes, I learn everything in the world back then. I used to play the guitar, too, and sing like my boy. But, you know, when I have my baby I forget all about it. Because I feel so sad, and I don't feel like doing it again. I forget everything, but I used to play and sing. Then I learn almost everything.

My grandmother was a midwife; she did it for all the family. She learn it from her mother, and when I was a girl she let me watch. I also help with the animals. The first baby I deliver by myself was when I was fourteen years old. My grandmother went to deliver another lady about forty miles from home, and my aunt was expecting. My grandmother asked her, "How do you feel?"

My aunt say, "Oh, I feel OK. Don't worry about me, I won't have my baby until next week."

As soon as my grandmother went from home, she start feeling sick, and I was with the sheep. Then one of my sisters went for me, and she stayed with the sheep until I came back, so I deliver my first baby. When I was fourteen.

And when my grandmother came back, she said, "Where's Petra?"

They say, "She's in the room."

"Did she have her baby?"

"Yes."

"Who did it?"

"Jesusita."

"Oh, that's good," she says. She was so proud of me. Then my grandmother starts letting me help her. Everytime she have one, I help. I didn't was scared nor nothing.

I always said when I was a little girl that I want to be a nurse or a midwife, but I didn't have the chance to be a nurse. I didn't finish my school, just the eighth grade. So, I be a midwife, and I like it. I'm so happy all the time. It doesn't bother me when they need me any time, day or night.

Oh, I wish I was back on that time, days on the ranch, days when I was young. And I don't care if I have to work day and night. 'Cause look at my hands. They are not hurt, no broken bones, nothing, no. And I even used to ride, to ride on the bucking cow. Small calves. I used to ride them for fun. Sometimes I fall down, but I don't care. I have a good time.

Young Adulthood in Trujillo

MY TROUBLES START when I'm twenty-three years old. I get pregnant with my boyfriend. I tell him, and he says, "I don't care, I don't care if you are. I don't want to get married with you."

I say, "OK, then, OK. I do it by myself; I won't bother you." So I never talked to him again, never, never, and I don't like him; I hate him.

I told him, but I didn't tell anybody in the house. When they notice me, they were asking this, that, that, and that, and they try to scare me. "You have to say what's the matter with you, you're getting fat." Because I wasn't fat; I was thin.

And I say, "No, nothing, nothing."

But I was getting bigger and bigger so that my daddy went one night to my grandma's house, and he said, "Who is the father of that baby?"

She say, "I don't know." 'Cause I didn't want to tell them.

It's hard on me 'cause everybody treats me, I don't know how to say. They treat me different. They get mad with me, everybody, everybody in the house. And there's nothing I can do.

I couldn't do anything. I tried to run away once, but I didn't know where I was going. I was just trying to go to the mountains, I think. It was night, and my sisters feel me get up out of our bed. They wake up too and say, "What are you going to do?"

"I'm running away."

They say, "If you're running away we're going with you."

They don't want to let me go alone, so I decide to stay. I don't run away, but I pray on the woods where I was taking care of the sheep, crying in the woods, and ask my Lord to take me with Him, 'cause I want to die, I was so ashamed. I was praying and praying to take me with Him. Day and night. But He didn't; I'm still here, thanks to Him. He didn't want me that time; He wants me on this world. My time came, and I had a hard labor 'cause I was scared. That's why, that's why I know when the ladies I deliver are scared, from myself. I stay Monday all day and all night holding that baby. I didn't want to do anything. All I want to do is die. That's what I want to do, die. "Dear Lord, I want to die, take me with you." While I'm having that baby my grandmother yells at me and says I am bad and calls me names, and my daddy didn't want to do anything with me anymore. Yes, oh, they were so mad at me; that's why I was so scared. But my Lord didn't take me and next day, Tuesday morning at six, I have my boy. My grandmother deliver him, and he's a big baby, eleven pounds, near that.

It's real hard for me after my Ernesto born. Everyday, everyday they say, "I don't know why you do this. You don't have anything to do with that. Why did you do it?" Oh, everyday, everyday, and I'm ashamed; I feel ashamed. That's the truth.

I feel so ashamed, and when I remember that, I say, "Oh, Lord, I don't know why I did that." Because if you have a mistake you don't want to do it, but I don't know why. I don't know, because I wasn't a bad girl. No, I wasn't.

And, you know, back then we had the *dieta*. It's forty days when they take care of you after a baby. They don't let the mothers eat too many things; just a few things, *atole*, a drink made of corn meal, and meat, lamb meat and steer meat and chicken, and not too many foods, no. If they eat meat, they eat at noon but not in the morning nor at night, no heavy foods at night. And the mothers don't go out until fifteen days, with eight days in bed.

But when I have Ernesto my family didn't care about me. They didn't let me have the dieta. They make me get up, and they send me out. "You can go work, you can do this, you can do that," they say to me. They make me go out in the rain and work like usual, and they didn't help me wash diapers, they didn't. No, they didn't care about me. I'm sorry to tell that, but that's the way I go.

And, you know, I ate everything, even what you're not supposed to when you have a baby. I eat green chili, corn like we used to eat it, even though they say green chili is bad when you have a little one. I eat everything, watermelons and everything. Once my grandmother say, "Who eat this chili?"

"I did."

"Why?"

"It won't hurt me as much as it can hurt me working outside the way you make me." And she didn't say anything back. Yes, I eat even what I wasn't supposed to. You know why? Because I was so hurt, I didn't care about me anymore.

And when my Ernesto was born I didn't have clothes for him. I didn't have the things he needs. But a nurse, Olive Nicklin, went to visit the school, and the teacher told her about me. So she went to my house and visit me, and she said, "Jesusita, do you need something?"

And I told her, "No." That's why I told her, 'cause I was ashamed.

And she said, "I hear that you need some clothes for your baby."

And I told her, "Yes, and for me too."

So she didn't say anything. Next day she came on a truck, and, oh, she gave me a lot of things, so many that I couldn't use for two years. I like her, and I never forget that, never. She brings me a blanket, sheets and pillowcases, and underwear for me, nightgowns, and aprons, and clothes for Ernesto. I was so happy. And now I give clothes to other ladies when they need them 'cause I remember.

Yes, it was hard for me at home then. My grandma and daddy wouldn't let me go to the dances after Ernesto was born. They didn't let me go to mass. When I ask them, when I ask my grandmother, "May I go to mass?"

"No. Don't you see what you did? Ain't you ashamed to go face the people?" So I stop, I never ask.

Once I ask her again, "May I go to the dance?" Ernesto was two years old.

She said, "No, nobody likes you; nobody's going to dance with you." So, I feel sorry, and I start crying, and I went to the mountains. I didn't care anymore, no.

And when Ernesto was three years old my friends went to see me where I was taking care of the sheeps, and they were having a big barbeque right up in Alta Vista, about eight miles from where we lived. When they were going, they said, "Jesusita, are you going to dance tonight?"

"No, they don't let me."

"Come on, try and go."

So you know what I said? "Yeah, sure I'm going tonight. I'm going tonight, and nobody's going to stop me."

You see, when they say to me, "Do this," I don't feel like doing it; but if I say, "I'll do this," I'll do it. I don't know why.

And when I go home and get the sheep to the corral and lock them there, I went to put water to warm to have a good bath and get my clothes and hang it and my shoes. I had my high heels and my stockings and everything, because I used to keep everything.

And my grandmother ask me, "What are you doing?"

"Get ready for the dance," I say.

"No ma'am, you don't have to go," she says.

"I'm going, and I'm going."

She looked at me and got mad. "If your daddy comes tell him like you're telling me."

"Sure, of course I'll tell him." And he was standing on the door hearing us. And I told him, "Yes, yes, Papa. I'm going to dance tonight, and don't tell me not to go because I'm going."

And I didn't feel sorry for them. I know what I did. And he didn't say anything. My grandmother tells me, "If you're going to dance take your little *muchacho*, your baby."

And that's the first thing my daddy do for me. He get Ernesto by his hand and takes Ernesto to his house, and he didn't say anything. So, that makes me feel that he's going to take care of Ernesto. So I went to the dance, and my grandmother was real mad. But I went to the dance.

My sisters go with me, but when I get to the hall and hear the music I feel so sad, and I tell my sisters, "No, I'm not going in. I don't feel like going in."

And my sisters say, "If you're not going in, and you're going back home, we're going with you."

So I said, "No." They don't have to lost this dance for me. So, I went in, and I start dancing the same thing like before my baby. And people didn't ask me anything.

They didn't say, "Why did you not come? I heard that you had a baby." No. Nobody ask me nothing. Oh, they were just so glad to see me. They liked me. It's a good memory, real good.

Later I have more sadness. I get pregnant again, and I have my daughter by myself because when I tell my grandma that I was sick that way, that I was pregnant, she say, "I don't care. If you're sick, that's up to you. You don't have any obligation to be like that, so, that's up to you. You have your baby alone."

She didn't care. I'm sorry to say that, but she didn't care. Even though others have babies alone, my grandma wouldn't forgive me. But I wasn't scared. No, I wasn't afraid, and when I'm in labor, I get my bed ready and everything ready, scissors, the string, the afterbirth pan, everything ready. I fix my bed, so when I kneel down to put the sheet down on the mattress, the water broke, and the baby came. Just right away. I didn't feel pain.

Oh, I had good luck with my daughter, and she weigh ten-and-a-half pounds. And when I see, like that, I see a girl with red hair and blue eyes. Like a doll. I named her after my grandmother; I name her Dolores. I was happy for my baby, for my girl, but not happy too because of all my troubles. So I say to myself, no more, that's all. No more babies.

In those years when you get in trouble, you don't have any place to go. No place to go. Just to stay there and get what they do with you. Sometimes I sit at the table, and they start talking this, talking that, and so sometimes I didn't eat. My grandmother and my daddy go on and on to me, but not my grandfather. My grandfather was nice, so nice to me.

Once my daddy had a party on December 24, and he invite everybody. I think he do that to hurt me. He invite everybody and not me, and, you know, when he sent one of his kids to tell my grandfather to go to the party, you know what my grandfather said? "No. If Jesusita doesn't go, I don't go either. I have enough for her and me." And he didn't go.

When I heard that I cried. I tell him, "Thanks, Grandfather. You are the only one that treats me good." And my grandfather tells me that the family has other things to feel bad about; they shouldn't just feel mad at me.

But my grandfather died, and when he died I didn't know what to do. He was the only one who treated me fine, the only one, and then I was really alone. Then my grandmother tells me she can't have me in her house, to get out and take my babies. To make my own living.

I start crying, and my daddy says, "Don't cry, you can stay with me."

And I told him, "No, I'm not used to live with you, with my stepmother and you mad at me all the time. With you so, so mad."

So he told me, "Where do you want to build your house?"

And I show him this place; I liked that place because it's on a little hill, and I always like to live on a hill. The trees are growing there now. There were too many little trees like those then, and I cut them down. I clean all around the place.

I went down the canyon, at my daddy's ranch, and cut down the trees for the wood for my house. And I hollow my wood and chop it and make a big pile for winter. I carry the wood back on my back, and Ernesto was about four years old, and he help me with one or two pieces of wood. He always goes with me to carry the wood. Always. Sometimes he cried, and I didn't know why. Maybe he got tired. I can say that now, I think he was tired, but I didn't know it then; I was young, too. I had two kids to take care of, my house to build, and all my farming and everything. But I knew how to build my house because my daddy built his house before, and I learn from him 'cause I help all the time.

I had a few things that belonged to my mother for furniture 'cause my grandma keep them for me. The other furniture I build. I remember I make Ernesto's little chair, high chair, and I make the chair to train him from wood in an old box.

And I make my garden near the mill, the windmill, and I have my animals. I have six cows of my own, and I have goats and sheeps of my own. They went to pasture in my daddy's place, but they are mine.

Yes, I had my animals, but some times were still hard, real hard. And, you know, they don't care. They don't care if I have something to eat or not. Sometimes I only eat bread with water. I don't have anything else to eat. So I feel so disappointed and I cry and say, "Why?" I don't know why. Sometimes you make a mistake, you don't know how. I never ask them for help. No. I never ask nobody because I feel like they don't want to help me. I didn't have any help but God, that's all.

I am lonely then. I feel lonesome for too many people. There are other single mothers, though. At that time we were about three. We help each other. When we get together we talk and cry about those things. We said, "Oh, we were crazy; we don't know why we did it." But we were young, and we don't know no better.

Other people were OK to me. They were friendly, and they say, "I don't know what's the matter with your daddy. I don't know, because you help him a lot, and I don't know what's the matter with him." They didn't like him to do that, the way he treat me. And, you know, my sisters, they used to cry for me too. They feel bad for me.

But my daddy wouldn't speak to me. No. We live about this house, and he didn't say, "Hello, Jesusita" or "Good morning," nothing, and he didn't like my boy. My boy feels bad, and he cries and I cry.

But in about three years my daddy needs me, and he said, when I came from work in the evening, he says, "Jesusita."

I get scared; I say to myself, "What's the matter with him? Maybe he's mad or something."

He says, "I need you tomorrow; you have to help me in the field. We are going to pull our beans." Well, I went, so I worked with my family again.

And later, when my father was dying, he feel sorry for me. He said, "Jesusita, forgive me."

And I told him, "No, I forgive you long time ago. A long time ago." He didn't even talk with me for three years when I have Ernesto, but I forgive him.

If I had my mother, she wouldn't let them put me out like that. She would have helped me, but they didn't care for me, and I didn't have my mother. That's why I was put out. A father is different from a mother. He's different.

My grandma didn't treat other mothers alone like that, and there were many babies like that, many. She's nice to them others. She doesn't talk mean to them. I don't know why she hurt me so. Seems to me she hated me.

Now I feel sorry for those girls, real sorry for them 'cause I know, I know. When these girls that I take care of are alone, they cry and feel ashamed. I tell them, "Don't be ashamed, I go that way too." But I feel sorry for them, sometimes I cry with them. 'Cause I know, and I feel sorry for that little baby too. Back then they want to hurt me, and they didn't care; they hurt me and that's all.

Sometimes I think they never care, even before I have my babies. You know why, I used to work outside, taking care of the sheep and everything. Back then we're not supposed to get wet when you're in your period. Well, the girls don't care anymore; they always are getting wet and everything, but then they weren't supposed to. But my family didn't care about me. I get wet everywhere I was, and next month I didn't feel any pain nor nothing; it come on the right time. But they don't care; they make me stay in the rain.

And I was sixteen when I start my period. My grandmother was worrying about me. She says, "Why, Jesusita, you don't have your period? You are the oldest, and one of my daughters began when she was ten, and the other one began when she was twelve, and what's the matter with you? What kind of girl are you?"

And that makes me so ashamed, so ashamed because she

always asking me about it. And I don't know why she ask me so often. You know, when I was sixteen I start, and I start on a big rain, and it didn't hurt me.

When my grandma was dying she called, "Jesusita, come here." And I went to her. She says, "You know, I'm worried about you."

"Why?"

"Because when you are going to change, I think you're going to suffer too much because we never took care of you."

And I told her, "Don't worry. It's too late for you to worry about that." Isn't that so? It was late, but, thanks to God, I didn't have a hard time.

After my grandfather died, I ask her, "Who are you going to stay with, Grandma?"

She says, "My sons, not you."

But she didn't last too long with them. No, she went back to me. And I buy a little goat, and I have green chili, and I make tortillas, a good supper. When she came she said, "Oh, it smells good here."

And I told her, "Yes, come in. You can eat with me, too."

And she said, "I won't go back to my sons again. I will stay with you. If you want me to."

And I told her, "Yes, you're welcome." Because I never get mad with nobody. They hurt me, but I can't get mad with nobody.

It was hard raising my babies alone, but there was good, too. They were fat and healthy kids. I didn't wrap my babies; I didn't swaddle them like others did, 'cause they couldn't stand it. They wanted to move and stay out and would cry if I wrapped them, so I didn't.

Dolores crawled in four months old and started walking eight months old, and she have her teeth when she was six months old. Ernesto start walking when he was a year and thirty-two days. He was slower than Dolores, 'cause he was scared, and Dolores wasn't. If Dolores near a bench or something, she get that bench with her hands and try to stand up. She wasn't scared, no; she try hard until she learn how to walk.

When they were little I make my own things and my tables, and when they were crawling and going to touch my good things, I didn't let them. I teach them that they don't have to do that, so they don't. If they did sometimes I slap a good one, and I don't let them jump on my bed, either. No, I teach them good. When they eat and get something on their hands, I don't let them clean on their clothes. I teach them good, and they're good kids.

You know, I saw a book of proverbs. One makes me remember when I used to sleep with my kids. It's a saying we used to have. It says, *El que con niños se acuesta, amanece bien mojado.* He who sleeps with children wakes up sopping wet. It makes me laugh. I sleep with my children, but I always keep them away from me, so I won't get wet.

I teach my kids too many things. I teach my own kids the catechism and the rosary. I make them pray with me everyday or everynight, every time we have a chance, and I remember well when they make their first communion, Oh, they look so pretty; Dolores dressed all in white.

We build a convent for the priest to live in. I used to wash the priest's clothes and to take care of the church, everything, and I like to help the sisters. One year we have two sisters over there, living in Don Miguel's house, and I help them after school, twice a week, I help. I know how to teach the kids catechism, but in Spanish, not in English. They never use English, no.

And I help when we build the new church. The old one was falling down. Don Miguel Anaya gives property for the new church, and we bring the stones and cement them. We make dances, dinner to sell for the church. We make something and raffle it to help the church, and finally we get a good new church.

But, oh, when I see the church now; those weeds and everything over there. Nobody cleans there. There's no more Jesusita. No, no more Jesusita to take care of it. No curtains on the windows. No more.

But I work hard for the church back then, but when the bishop went there to confirm the kids, you what what Mr. Anaya said? "They're not to confirm your kids, Jesusita."

"Why?" 'Cause I used to clean the church, wash the

priest's clothes and *las manteles del altar*, the altar cloth, and clean everything. And I ask him, "Why."
"Because you're not married."
And I didn't tell him anything, but when I get to the priest's room Mr. Anaya was with him, and I told the priest, "Well, I don't think I see you tomorrow."
He said, in Spanish, "We won't see you and your kids tomorrow? Why, Jesusita?"
"Because Mr. Anaya said that you are not going to confirm my kids because I'm not married."
The priest say, "Oh, Mr. Anaya, you can't say that. No sir, you have the right like everybody else, Jesusita."
I feel good then, and I bring my kids and they confirmed, but I was angry at Mr. Anaya. And, you know, he's got a big bunion, a big hump, on the back of his neck. You know what I used to tell the girls, my friends? "Mr. Anaya have the bunion, the big hump, because he carries everybody's sins, everybody's baddest things on his neck." And we all laugh and laugh.
Yes, the kids grow good. I remember them playing around the house, running and making noise and playing in the grass, and I remember them going to school. They came on the bus to school.
Our neighbor, Gregorio, used to teach Ernesto how to play the guitar, when he was nine or ten. Ernesto is good, like my grandfather was. My grandfather used to play the guitar, the violin, and the accordian. That's why I learn to dance and everything, and Ernesto learns to play good too.
I was lonesome by myself sometimes, and sometimes I think of marrying somebody else. I had a friend, a good guy 'cause I knew him since I was a little girl. He was older than me, not too much, but he was older.
And one day I was working in the bean fields when my friend comes to me and says, "Jesusita, I want to marry you."
I say, "What about my kids?"
But he told me that he don't want my kids because he wasn't the father.
So I told him, "OK, that's OK with me; I don't love you. I was trying to make you a good wife, but no, I don't want

you." Because I work too hard to support my kids, and so I told him, "Forget it, don't ask me anymore. Never." So that's why I don't want to get married with nobody, and, you know, he's already dead. And he die single, and he could have had a good wife. I didn't get angry with him, but I tell him, "Don't bother me anymore, never." He didn't.

My sister Soledad got married back then, and she and her husband build a new house near mine. It is big and white and so pretty. Soledad plants flowers all around it and is proud.

When my Dolores is four my sister Ramona gets pregnant without marrying. My daddy gets mad, and he blames me for that. He says, "That's why, because you have Ernesto and Dolores she thinks that's OK with me for her to have another one." No, they don't have to blame me, but they blame me; my grandma blame me, too.

And my daddy tells Ramona to go out. He says, "You know where to go, get out of my house." And Ramona got sick; she faint, fell on the floor.

And my stepmother jumped on me, too, but I answer my stepmother; I didn't answer my daddy, but I answer her. I told her, "You don't have anything to do with me, and you better shut up. You don't boss me." I jumped to her, too.

So we build a house for Ramona and her baby boy, Ben. The house is near to mine, and we help each other those years. We're close to each other, but my sister is sick since Ben is born, ever since my daddy kicked her out. She gets worse everyday, more and more. She is always sad and cries a lot. I think she didn't want to live. She never say nothing, but I think she didn't want to live. I try too many things for her, but I couldn't do anything. I try herbs and something like that. I know they're good, but they didn't help.

We take her to the doctors, but the doctors didn't help either. Now that I see too many things, I don't want to say the doctors don't know anything in those years, but the doctors know more now, have more experience, and they study too much, and they found how people get sick. Then the doctors didn't know what happened with my sister, and she got worse.

Finally, Ramona calls me to her and tells me, "I know I'm going to die, but Ben is yours. Don't let him go to anywhere else. It's yours, and raise him and teach him. He's a good boy."

Ben's six years old when Ramona dies. He's very sad, and all the time I find him here under that tree behind the house crying for his mother, so he makes me cry too. So now I have three kids to raise, and I raise them, but I feel bad to bury Ramona and be away from her after so many years. Now the cross is broken on her grave, and it's not pretty anymore. Well, it's sad to see that. Nobody's there, that's why, but I'll have my Ernesto make a cross, and we'll fix it again.

Sometimes we have hard times back then, me and my three kids. I didn't have any welfare because they never used to give any welfare, but they give those commodities, like food stamps now. The truck went to Trujillo, but I never got any, so I take my aunt and two of my neighbors to get them in my daddy's wagon and team. When we got there, I told them, "Do you need any help?"

They say, "Yes, jump up here."

So he gives me the hand, and I jump in the truck and help him 'cause the packets have the people's name, and when I get down from there, you know what? I get more than nobody else because I help him, a big load, and I get them every month.

I do lots of jobs to support my kids. I used to work on the fields. I used to work everywhere; cleaning house, washing clothes, ironing clothes for somebody else, and hard work, but I raise my kids.

And I went to work in Colorado on the fields. My daddy moved there, later when it's getting too dry in Trujillo. My daddy writes to me and he says, "Come, Jesusita, I need make a good winter. Come and work here." So we go. We go for two summers and work the crops.

It is hard work. It's warm weather over there, and you have to work all day, long rows. Oh God, it's hard. We get up at four and start here about five or six in the morning, and you came back to the same place by the same time in the evening. We stay at night with my daddy, and we work in the same place all summer. When we finished with this the other thing is ready. The kids work with me on the onions, lettuce, and beets. I used to work in the fields in Trujillo pulling beans and cutting corn, everything, so I was used to working in the fields and know how. And we pick carrots, tomatoes, watermelons. To pick them, they were heavy, you can't pick just one or two. They're too heavy, so you can carry them where the truck can get them. And cantaloupes, lettuce, and pickles. We pick them all.

We work hard, and the kids help pretty good. They don't complain too much. Yes, we got tired, but we got to work too. But I never get too tired when I was young. Never, and nothing hurts me. I didn't get sore nor anything. Oh, sometimes I cut my hands; it's unusual, but I never get too tired. I don't know why, but never, and that's a good gift. God gave me that.

We work with lots of people, too many people from everywhere. And they tell us about other places, about Mexico, Red River, and Tucumcari, but I never deliver babies when I'm there. No, 'cause nobody knows me there.

My daddy says, "If you live here you get rich. You get rich, Jesusita. Look at those people; everybody is pregnant." But I never tell those pregnant women; I never tell them that I'm a midwife. I don't know why; I just never tell them.

And when we come from Colorado, back to Trujillo, I buy my children enough supplies to go to school for all the winter. Everything, you know, pencils and tablets and clothes and enough food, enough food for them.

I used to deliver babies, lots of babies, from a long time before we go to Colorado until along time after. There were four of us midwives in Trujillo, Canutita Crespin and Petra Archuleta and Dona Lujana, and they were glad when I start because they were getting old like me now. They say, "Oh, that's good, Jesusita. You're going to be in our place." And they talk to me, how to do this and how to do that and how to change the bed and everything. They teach me 'cause they like it when I start to be a midwife. Oh, yes, and later, when I get my diploma, they never do it again. They call me to deliver their families; they were just watching me, and that makes me proud.

I used to go far to deliver babies. The father of the baby comes to get me. I go lots on horseback and sometimes on a wagon or car, but most of the time on horseback 'cause I like it better. I don't like the wagon, and I told them, "No, don't bring the wagon, bring two horses. It's easy because you can make a shortcut." Sometimes I go twelve miles, sometimes three, sometimes one mile, and sometimes thirty-four or forty miles, but that far only in a car.

My daddy taught me about a midwife who was murdered a long time ago. My daddy was about sixteen years old when it happen. Two men came and tell her that they need her in Santa Rosa, so she went with them that way. They never get there, and she asks them, "Where is the house?"

"No here, not here, not here," they answer.

And they take her to the woods and hang her and hurt her in bad ways and kill her. In about three days her people are worried and worried, and so they go out and look for her, and a rancher finds her hanging on a tree.

So it's dangerous to go out because sometimes you go out when you don't know that guy who comes to get you, and you don't know if you can trust him or not. But you have to go, and any hour, night or day. I have to go, and every midwife, every midwife has to go, and you never know where you are going or what it is going to be like 'cause you don't know if they are lying or what.

Everybody treats me OK, though, except for one time. Two boys come to my kitchen door that time, and one of the boys says, "Are you Jesusita?"

"Yes."

"Well, my wife is going to have a baby, and she told me to take you there."

"Who is your wife?" And he doesn't know what to say.

So I say, "No, that's not true mister, go away." And I close my door.

It wasn't true, no. Because if a lady's going to have a baby that man comes in a hurry, and he says what he has to say.

This boy didn't sound good, and I'm glad I didn't go with him. If I'm ever afraid on the way to a delivery, I pray. I pray on the way to help the lady.

Once a nurse comes to Trujillo to teach a class for mothers. That nurse's name is Edith Rackley, and I still know that lady. We are friends. I go to the class, and she says, "Can anyone here read these papers to the other mothers?" And I say, "Sure, I can read them for us." And she says, "Thanks" and is glad to have my help.

Sometime later I go to her and tell her I'm a midwife, and I want to take a special class they have for midwives, a class in Las Vegas the nurses have.

Then we come here to town in Las Vegas, and we stay about fifteen days, and the government pays everything, the trip, the board and room, everything. There are about thirty to forty-five women from different places, from Los Lunas, Santa Rosa, Wagon Mound, and only me from Trujillo.

They teach us many things. One of the nurses, Mrs. Ordonias, she was about fifty or fifty-two years, and she told me that I should have my nails short, clean, because we have to show our nails, but I never use my nails; I never let them grow. I can't use them if I do.

My grandmother teach me to wear my apron years ago, but the nurses talk more about how to use it. And now my neighbors know when my patient is going to have her baby because I get ready and put my white apron, and they see it and say, "Oh, pretty soon the baby's coming." They know it's near to come because of my apron.

The class had many interesting things. I didn't like to miss the meetings nor the movies because they teach us with good movies, movies of natural birth and other kinds of birth and D and C's and bad diseases like gonorrhea. They taught us that's why the patients have to go to the clinic and have a blood test, so that way they know if they have something wrong, and if they have something wrong it hurts the baby. But some of the patients don't believe on those things, but I do, I do believe. They're supposed to have a blood test before the baby born. If they don't have their blood test before, they are supposed to go to the hospital as soon as they get out so they can be checked.

After fifteen days of the class we have a test and have to answer twelve questions, and we can only miss two or three. I didn't miss any. Then we have a little dinner to see which one gets the diploma and a pin. I got my pin, my home nursing pin.

Then we form a midwife club. We come together to have meetings and to get supplies the nurses give us to help with our deliveries, and we have officers. We pay two dollars a year. That money is for the parties, for the coffee, cookies, and small sandwiches, and at Christmas we fix our Christmas tree, and at the clinic we have a special room for our meetings.

Later, after I came to Las Vegas, the midwives help the clinic. About 1960 it happens. The old clinic, then, was so crowded, and everybody wants a new one with more room. But the people who run Las Vegas don't pay attention to the nurses, and so we midwives help the nurses out.

We get lots of papers saying we need a new building, and we take those papers around to our friends, and our friends sign the papers 'cause everybody wants a new clinic.

And they build the clinic and make an open house when it is finished. They have refreshments and everything, and everybody is happy, the nurses and doctors and midwives too. It's a beautiful clinic with X-rays and everything. Yes, we helped each other then.

Life in Las Vegas

I LIVED IN TRUJILLO with my three kids until Ernesto was ready to start high school. There were good neighbors and everything in Trujillo, but the school just goes to eighth grade, and I want my kids to go to high school.

I wanted to go to high school myself, but they didn't want to bring me here. I used to talk and talk to them about it, but they say, "No, we can't. That's all, we can't." So I stop asking them, but it's important that Ernesto and Dolores and Ben go.

So in 1952 I sell the wood in my house and pay a neighbor to move me to Las Vegas. First I move to New Town, Mr. Pena's, and then I move near here and rent there too. Then later I buy this place of land and build my house.

When I first came here I washed for people and ironed and cleaned houses and cleaned doctors' offices too. I wash for people on the wash board and wash tub, with my hands like I always did in Trujillo. Then one of the people I work for, she found me washing on the wash board, and she says, "Jesusita, why didn't you tell me. Oh, no, no. It's too hard for you."

So she takes me to her store that she runs, and she has me pick out a washing machine, electric iron, and a ironing board, and then she uses her truck to bring them to my house, and oh, it was so easy. So, I pay for them by doing her washing, cleaning her house, making her tortillas, taking care of her kids so she can go to a dance, many things. Yes, back then I have to clean too many houses, and I have to wash the floors on my hands and knees. It was hard work then; now everything is easy. They have vacuum cleaners, and you are not kneeling down. Dolores helps me so much during the times when I work in Las Vegas. She takes all the care of our house while I work on my jobs. She's a good girl and doesn't get into trouble.

One day I quit cleaning and I went to work at the parachute factory on the plaza. There were 475 of us, mostly ladies and a few men and our three bosses. Our three bosses were men. I work there eleven years, for a long time, until they close the factory.

I do many things at the factory. I rip, I cut, I sew, I darn. I'm the only one who darns. One day my boss said, "I'm going to train you, Jesusita, so you can darn the parachutes when they snap."

And I told him, "You don't have to train me. I am trained."

So he says, "Are you?"

"Yeah."

"Who trained you?"

"My grandmother, with socks with a little hole in the cloth."

So he gave me a piece of rag and a very, very small needle with a long eye, and I used three threads from the parachute, and I made the sample, and he likes it.

Then in about two or three weeks there was a parachute jumper from Albuquerque, and he wants to jump fifty or seventy-five times with the same parachute and needs it fixed, and he brings that parachute to us. He says, "Is there anybody who can fix this?"

"Yes, I have one. I have a lady who can fix it." So I fixed it, and we sent it back to Albuquerque.

At the factory my boss asked me one day, "What is your short name? Because Jesusita is too hard for me."

And I told him, Jessie because when I was in school sometimes they call me Jessie. So at the factory everybody called me Jessie. I'm Tita, Jesusita, and Jessie.

They like my work at the parachute factory. When my boss asks me to stay two or three hours after work, overtime, I never say no; I never say no. Sometimes I didn't get off work until 11:00 at night. Yes, and then I have to go at 6:00 in the morning, but I was young and strong.

Sometimes I would leave to deliver babies, and one time somebody from another town came to get me almost as soon as I go to work. So, I asked my boss if I could go, and he said, "Go ahead."

I wasn't at the lady's too long, the birth came a little fast, but it was far, and when I came back my time card wasn't there to be punched like the others. Everybody calls me and says, "Jesusita, they're going to send you home; they're going to fire you. You were gone too long."

I said, "Well, I can't help it," and then I turned and looked to the window where my boss was in the office, and he called me to him with his hand.

And I feel bad. You know how it is when you need the money, when you need to work. So I tell my friends, "Goodbye, girls."

Then my boss said, "Come here, Jessie. Where did you go?"

I don't know, I was afraid to tell him the truth because I said, "If I tell him the truth he won't give me any more work."

So, he asks me, "Did you punch your card?"

"No, I didn't."

"Why?"

"Because you got it here."

"Who told you that?"

"Nobody, but I think that you got it here."

So he told me, "You know what, Jessie, I have to send a shipment tonight, and I need eighty special pieces for the harness."

And I told him, "I can make them for you by this evening."

He said, "Oh, no. I don't think you can. That's too much. I bet you some coffee that you can't."

I said, "Oh, I can; I can."

"OK, OK," he says. "Here is your card, punch it and go to

work on those pieces. I can't send you home because I like your work; you do everything I tell you."

Then I go back to my work, and everybody said, "What did he say?"

"Oh, nothing, nothing." So I didn't pay any attention to them, and then I make 125 of the harness pieces, by 6:00 in the evening, 125.

Then the boss called me in, and he said, "How many did you make?"

"One hundred and twenty-five."

"I don't believe you; I won't pay you," he said, but he was joking with me.

And the next day he gave me $5.00 'cause he'd bet with me. He said, "Here is your $5.00 for the coffee and something else."

I still go out to deliver babies, and one day he says, "Jessie, I want to know, why do you go out so often."

I don't know what he thinks of me, so I get my license out of my pocket and show it to him.

"Why didn't you tell me? I was ready to fire you, to send you back three times."

"Well, if you send me home I can look for another job."

"No, that's OK, and you can go out when they need you." So, he never bothers me again. When somebody goes to the office and asks for me, my boss goes and stands by me and says, "Somebody needs you better; you have another baby."

And they let the ladies who are pregnant work, to the last minute, and you know what he says, "You don't have to quit; here is Jesusita." And when they're to lift a heavy box or something, he says, "No, don't do it," and he looks for something easier for them to do.

When we work at the parachute factory we had parties, too, for Christmas. Our boss makes us take everything away from the tables, and the tables were so long, more bigger than this house, 'cause parachutes are too big, for the jeeps or another load they throw from the air. They put food for our party on those long tables, and oh, we have everything to eat on that party. He gave us that party, and when we came out from the party there was a truck load with him, candies and turkeys. He was nice to us.

But he dies of a heart attack. He was playing ball, and he dies before he gets to the hospital. We cry and cry that day. The row where the people go and visit him at Roger's Mortuary was so long. He was wrapped on a white cloth, white material, wrapped from his head to his feet. They said that they're going to burn him in Utah where he lives. They burn the body, and they put the ashes in a little box. They never do that way here, never.

Yes, we had a good boss in those days, but I worked hard too. I didn't get much sleep back then, but I didn't get tired. Well, you know, a little tired, but I never get lazy nor nothing. I'm not lazy now neither, but I am a little tired. Well, I'm getting old; years make the difference.

I did lots back then. While I was working at the parachute factory I get ready to build my house, the house I live in now. I was working there, and then when we get off, about 4:00 or 4:30, I come here and work on my house. When it gets dark I build a fire, so I can see to work.

There wasn't nothing here then, no electricity, no water. So I and Julia, my friend, and Mrs. Durán, my neighbor, we get together, the three of us, and we go to the electric plant and ask for light. They say, "Yes, we give it to you if you dig the big holes for the poles, because we are too busy to dig them."

So Ben and one of my nieces, Agapeta Trujillo, dig my two holes for me, and Julia paid them to dig the two for her, and Mrs. Durán paid them, too. So in about three days we have light here.

Then we ask for the water, too. We have to pay thirty-five dollars each, and if somebody opens the line, that money come back to me and to everyone. They turn our money back; that was good.

You know, the men, they won't do anything. They say, "Oh, no, you won't get anything." But they don't care, but we women do it. We try it and do it. Sometimes women do things better than them, better than men.

You know, I won prizes at dances, when I first come to town. My sister, Soledad, was living here, and one night she says, "Let's go to dance, a dance here in Boulevard Street and San José Hall."

I told her, "No, I don't like to go to dances here in town." 'Cause I don't know, I was used to going to the ranch. When I have time I go back to the ranch and dance over there. Not just me, we get together, three or four families, and we go in a bus or in a truck or something back to Trujillo, and we have a good time back there.

But Soledad says, "Come on, let's go. Do you know why I want you to go? To win the prizes because Miguel Archuleta and Anita, his wife, win the prizes all the time."

So I told her, "OK, I'll go," and that's when I start going to dances here. They are just the same, just the same as in Trujillo, and I have a good time here, too. So the first piece we danced was a polka and then a cuadrilla, a square dance in English. There were judges to decide, and everybody say, "Come on, Jessie. Come on, Jessie. Make it, you have to make it, to win the prize." So I won the prize, and I feel very happy.

Once, during the second world war, there was another barn dance that was to have old-fashioned clothes. So everybody invites me at the factory, and I sew my own dress. I make it like the dresses on my grandma's and mother's picture. I buy the material, and I make it in a little while 'cause I used to sew. But they used high shoes with a string back then, and I need those shoes. So I go to what was the Martinez store then. Manuel Martínez was the owner, and we know him very well. We told him, "Come on, Don Manuel, find me a pair of shoes; I need green."

And he says, "OK. Let's go down the cellar, maybe I have some down there." And I found two pairs. It was a long dress, and I had my shoes, and I comb my hair and put a bow, a rainbow in it, and I won the prize on the old-fashion dress.

Those were good times, and, you know, they never fight back then at the dances. They didn't get drunk, nor nothing like now.

I can still dance. My son dances with me; he likes to dance a polka or a waltz with me. Oh, he's a good dancer. On one of my birthdays, not long ago, on March 26, my son told me, "Come on Tita; let's go to Frank's tonight." So I get ready and went with them, with some friends and Ernesto, and I didn't have a chance to sit down. Everybody invites me to dance. As soon as I get in, everybody. Everybody likes to dance with me, and I don't get tired, no. I'm strong, that's right, and my feets don't hurt me. I don't get sore, my legs nor nothing.

The next day, somebody said, "Oh, I'm so sore; I dance too much last night. Are you sore?"

"No, I'm not, no. I'm fine."

My boy decides to go to the army when he's twenty. He takes the exam and passes it, and he likes to go because he wants to see too many places. He says, "Don't cry, Mama, don't cry. I want to know all the places I can, and I don't have that money. But the government will pay."

Then he goes to Germany, when he's twenty-two. Oh, I got so many pictures from him, so many pictures. I have two albums when Ernesto was in the army. When he went to Germany he made pictures on the ship. I have all the letters and everything. He was happy back then and that makes me happy.

Dolores and Ernesto and Ben all get married later. Dolores is happy but has a small wedding and so does Ben, but Ernesto says to me, "I want a big wedding. I'm not a widow nor an old man." And he does have a big wedding, at Immaculate Conception. My daddy was there; he was still strong and happy, and it was a fine day.

Then I have grandchildren. Ernesto has two, Consuelo and Steve, and Dolores has three, Michael and Erwin and Martha. I deliver them all, and they start staying with me when they're really little, everyday.

Ben marries a woman who has three kids. He has two stepdaughters who are older and a stepson named Dwight. Then he and his wife have another boy, Randy. At first they live in Albuquerque, and then they move to Pueblo. Ben works in the sky with steel.

Once Dolores and her husband move to Albuquerque, but they couldn't stay there because the kids cry a lot for me. I went to visit one time, and they want to come back with me. The next day I come home, but I cry too when I get away. And soon they have to move back because the kids are crying, oh so much, for me. You see, I missed them because they are near; they are raised with me.

I have many good times with my grandchildren. When they were little I dressed Consuelo and Martha alike. In the same color, in the same clothes, and then when they're all pretty I take them to mass with me.

Consuelo got married not so long ago, and I dressed her for her wedding. And I tie them together with a black string, Consuelo and her groom. You know why I tie them, because they want to steal the bride, take her away, and hide her. Then they pass the hat to get some money to bring the bride right back. It's a new way; they make it just for fun. And it's true, we have a good, good time.

My sister Soledad lived here in Las Vegas when my grandchildren were little, but when Soledad is forty-nine she gets real sick. She has diabetes and high blood pressure, and a vein breaks all over, all over her head. She gets blind and two days, it's over, and she dies. I miss her. She's my last full sister. There were eight of us born to my mother, and now I am the only sister left.

But there was my daddy. My sisters and I used to take good care of my daddy. We didn't let my daddy chop wood nor anything. Oh no, we treat him like a little boy, and we spoil him. We loved him, but when he moved to Colorado he works hard there because we weren't there.

The first time I went to La Junta to visit him, I found him chopping wood. So I get mad with my other sisters, my half sisters, and I ask for my daddy when I get to their house. I say, "Where is my father?"

"He's chopping wood," my stepmother told me.

"Why? He's not used to do it."

"Well that's with you, not with us." That's what she said.

So I put on my old clothes, because I always take my old clothes everywhere I go, my old shoes, my apron, and everything. My father didn't know that I was in the house, so I went out to the yard, and I call him, "Papa, here I am."

So he came and give me a kiss and a hug, and I told him, "Why are you chopping wood?"

"Because I don't have you here," that's what he told me.

And I feel sorry for him because he was getting old and working, like me now, the way I work now. I took better care of him than a boy would have done. Yes, I did.

But when my daddy's eighty-one years old, in 1965, he gets sick. He gets gangrene. It starts from the bottom of his feet, and they cut his legs, but he never complains. He take it so easy, and if you ask him, "Do you want to have something 'cause you feel bad?"

"No, I don't need anything; I'm OK."

But he lives just eight months. I am with him when he dies. Like I told before, he says, "Jesusita, forgive me for how I treat you when your babies born."

And I told him, "No, I forgive you long ago," and he dies.

When he dies I feel so bad. I take it so hard 'cause he was the last thing I have in the world. But when I'm home, and the people come to visit me and tell me that they are sorry for me, because everybody knows me, I feel better. When nobody came I was crying, and, oh, I don't know; I can't explain, but I need to have somebody here. Yes, I'm used to it, to having people. When I'm sad my friends come, and I feel better. Friends help. And now I am the oldest, of neighbors and relatives and everything; now there's just me.

So many things change over the years. Many things change in how we deliver babies. When I first be a midwife, some mothers give birth the old way; the way that's gone now. They squat down when they have their baby. They tie a little round stick on the string, on a little rope. Then they put the rope over the *vigas*, the beams in the ceiling. They put it over so it's like a handle for her, and she squats down and holds onto the stick. Oh, it helps. I like that way, and sometimes somebody hold her from the back. They hold her back against their leg so she doesn't fall over.

I deliver two that way, and one of them was my sister-in-law. I don't know why, but with her first baby, she kneels down, and she says, "I feel better that way." So kneeling down is not too hard. And another lady, she does the same thing. It helps. I don't know why they stop doing that way, why they start laying on their backs. I think because to squat down is an old-fashioned way.

And we used to do different with the placenta. As soon as

the placenta comes out you're supposed to take that placenta to some other room or to the bathroom, or take it out
and bury it right away. Because they say the mothers feel
bad when the placenta's in the room with them; they feel
cramps or sometimes upset.

You know, when that lady is having her baby, I'm praying,
but not loud. Praying for that lady to be OK, and for that
baby, 'cause I learn to pray from my grandmother. My grandmother says, "Pray when you have a patient, pray for her
and pray for that baby." So I learn everything. I pray in my
mind, not loud. I pray in my heart by myself. I always pray
for them, always.

I have paintings of the saints in the room I use for the
babies. My San Luis belonged to my great-grandmother and
is very old. During the deliveries I pray to those saints:

> San Martín de Porres,
> ayúdame que salga con bien.
> San Antonio, cuídalas.
> San Luis Gonzaga, cuídame
> asi tambien que salga todo bien.

It means:

> San Martín de Porres,
> help me that it comes out fine.
> San Antonio, take care of them.
> San Luis Gonzaga, take care of me
> also so everything will be all right.

And I learn how to baptize from my grandmother, too. I
baptize many. When the mothers think their baby is going
to die, they tell me, "Baptize my baby."

I know how to baptize, and I know how to pray, baptizing
that baby. I say, "I baptize you in the name of God, the Holy
Ghost, and the name of the Father and Son." And I put some
water on the baby's head, make a cross with the water, holy
water or any kind of water. If you have holy water, use it,
but any kind of water is blessed 'cause God blesses everything in the world.

Back then they used to wrap the babies. They used to

wrap their heads with a big handkerchief, a spare one, and put the handkerchief back behind the babies' necks so the babies can hold their heads. And now, no; they don't do it now. I think the babies are stronger now. They're bigger too, much bigger. I don't know why; but that's the way it is. They don't need any handkerchiefs now, and if you wrap the hands down to get them warm, soon the babies put their hands up. I guess the hospitals don't wrap the babies, and that makes the mothers think it is an old-fashioned.

Now if there are tiny babies, premature babies, they take them to the hospital and into the incubator, but long ago I had two babies, two-pound babies, and they grow; they're alive. One is a nurse at the hospital in Pueblo; that's my nephew. He weighed two pounds when he was born. He was only six months along. He didn't have nails, nor hair, nor nothing. Nothing, just a tiny little baby. And when he opens his mouth you don't hear any sound because he's too little to have sound yet.

We say, "We should take him to Las Vegas, to the hospital."

But his mother says, "No, by the time you get there my baby will die." So we don't take him, but she is scared all the time and would say, "My baby's going to die; he's going to die." But they take care of him in a little box on the oven door, and they keep just a little piece of wood in the stove so to have low heat, for two months they do this. It is hard because at night one of them has to watch for several hours and the other one another hour, something like that. They feed him with a dropper, but he lives and is all grown now.

My grandmother teaches me how to take care of sick babies. She teaches me how to breathe in babies' mouths if they don't breathe themselves. I don't know if the other midwives know how to do that, but I know how.

After the baby's born back then they have the dieta. Remember the dieta's for forty days after the baby. This is time when the mothers are careful, and they don't eat too many things. They eat atole, steer meat, chicken, and lamb meat, and they make food like bread with lard. And they make like tortillas and doughlike turnovers, then open them and put them in the oven, and they roast them so tender and good. But they never eat tortillas, nor potatoes, nor beans, nor chili because they all nurse their babies then, and my grandma says that the beans are no food for the baby. They get too much gas with beans.

During the dieta the mothers stay eight days in bed, and they don't go outside until fifteen days, and then only if it's not windy or rainy. But not me, remember how they made me get up and work right away. But for the other mothers, they don't let them sweep nor wash, iron, neither sew. I don't know why. My grandmother used to say that if they sew it might hurt their eyes.

And they don't let them sleep with their husbands, no. She sleeps where the baby was and the man a little ways away, until forty days. After forty days the mother takes a bath and says to the man, "OK, it's all yours." But sometimes her period starts, so she has a little longer. With the dieta the mothers has some time to get OK.

Once I had a so sad thing happen with my friend. She was pregnant with her third baby, and her mother told her, "Why don't you ask Jesusita to deliver your baby?"

"Oh, no," she says, "I'd be embarrassed; I'm ashamed."

So they come to Las Vegas and take a midwife from here. My friend was about my age, and I was about thirty years old.

But she couldn't do it. She couldn't have that baby. A little arm came out and that arm stay all day, all day out, and the midwife didn't let her people know what's happening. But her family finds out, and they come for me. I come, and I wash my hands, and I see her.

I tell the midwife, "Why didn't you tell them that this happened to her?" I'm so angry with the midwife, she doesn't tell me anything.

And I get some olive oil and put it on that baby's arm and push the arm back. Then I get the patient on her side and hold that arm, and I straight the baby's head, and it come just right out. But she was dead; that baby was dead.

And the midwife wanted to go as soon as I get there, but I didn't let her. I told her, "No, you better wait. You're supposed to wait. If you take this lady to the hospital, you have to be with her, or if you call another midwife, you have to stay with her." Too many times I have to do that; I have to go too late. Why didn't she say early? That lady was my friend.

When we used to have so many midwives in Las Vegas, and they have a problem they used to call me. The families would say, "Go bring Jesusita."

And I would go and ask the midwife, "Why is she so delayed?"

"I don't know what's the matter with her," the other midwife would say. So, I'd wash my hands and examine that lady and find the water bag is hard.

And then I used to ask them, "Why, can't you tell me? Why?"

"No."

"Why didn't you break the water bag?"

"'Cause I don't know how." And then I break the water bag, and the baby come right out.

Sometimes, though, the mother dies when the baby is born, and then there is much sadness. If that happens the grandmother have to raise that baby. She milks the cows or a goat and puts the milk in the bottle. They use any kind of bottle. They clean it and use small nipples, not big ones like now. The grandmother raises the baby because they don't want to give that baby away. No.

Once in a while, somebody else in the family nurses that baby. I saw it in Red River. The mother dies, and they give the baby to her aunt, who was older. The aunt drinks some beer, and the beer helps her, and then she puts the baby to suck. When she starts doing that, everybody laughs at her, but in a few days the aunt has as much milk as if she was a young girl.

When I was about ten I saw something funny. When a baby was born his mother die, and the family ask my grandfather for a goat to milk for the baby. And, you know, that goat was like she was his mother. They'd wash the goat's udder, and the goat would come and stand across the cradle, and they would put that baby to feed. The goat would just stand still by herself, and the baby drinks from the goat, and they don't have to give the baby no more bottle.

The goat would sleep in the baby's room, and when that

baby got older the goat watched that baby. Everywhere the kid goes, the goat goes with him and don't let nobody to hurt him. So when he was four years old, they take the goat to my grandfather, and they want to buy that goat because the boy likes that goat, and the goat likes the baby, the boy. So my grandfather gives the goat to him, because the boy was crying for that goat. I don't blame him, the goat was like his mother.

My grandmother told me something a long time ago. She said, "Remember, Jesusita, if you're going to be a midwife for years, watch yourself, don't get scared. When those babies born, they're going to be more and more stronger."

And now, when I'm cleaning them some of them smile at me. Yeah, smile. Kids or my neighbors see that. Somebody has to be here with me, and they see those babies so smiley with me, smiley like a big baby. Or sometimes I'm going to clean the babies, and they get ahold of my apron with their hand. They're scared and want to hold on. They're bigger too than they used to be. A couple of pounds more. "Yes," I think. "Maybe my grandma was right."

Today I still deliver babies. The ladies come to me when they think they're pregnant. They go to public health too, for the tests. When she first comes I check to see if the baby's in good position. I check with my hands, by the way they feel. When the baby's a breech baby the head is up at the top.

I tell the lady the supplies she needs. She needs blankets and binders for the baby, diapers, olive oil, and things for the lady. And I have the string, tape, nylon for the cord on my own. I used to get them here at the clinic, but they don't have them anymore for me. And I have to buy my own gauze for the cord, because I'm an old-fashioned midwife. I learned that things from my grandmother, to take care of the cord and put a binder around it, and to put a binder around the patient too. Yes, it's old-fashioned.

You know, I can't use my rubber gloves. But I think doctors use them because they go from one infection to another, and they're scared they'll give that infection to a mother. But I wash my hands real good, with a brush, and I have short nails and everything.

When the mother's in labor she comes to my house, and I stay with her through it. Sometimes I go to her house, but mostly she comes to mine. And, thanks to God, everybody's satisfied with me.

They say, "Oh, you have so nice hands, smooth." I don't have smooth hands; I have hard hands, but they feel my hands are smooth. I don't touch them hard nor nothing. I touch them just gentle and pet them. It helps. They feel so good, and they say, "Oh, Jesusita, I love you."

And I talk with them and sometimes I make them laugh. Yes, they feel better, and sometimes I tell them, "Get up and sit here in the kitchen and talk with me. I'm going to make supper." Or dinner, or breakfast. And that way they feel better talking. We get their things out, and I say, "Stay here; don't worry. I'm here; I'm ready." They feel better that way.

But if you are mad with them, they don't feel good. No. They say to the midwife, "I mustn't come here." 'Cause I hear them sometimes, talking about the other midwives, but I look like that I don't hear nothing.

Some of the midwives got mad, though. I know that there was a midwife that used to slap them when they cry or get nervous, but she didn't last too long. They disqualify her. They took her certificate away because the people say at the clinic what kind of midwife she is. Now I get a license, and every year they send it from Santa Fe to me.

Sometimes the ladies cry during labor, 'cause it hurts. Some of them get mad too, like they're blaming me, and they say, "Don't touch me. Get away from here." But I know that's normal, sometimes. When I went to school I learned those things.

Sometimes they try to pinch you or scratch you, but, little by little, they calm. I never get mad with them; I tell them, "Don't scratch me, don't be like that. Don't blame me on that, that's your own fault," I say.

Sometimes they laugh, or sometimes they say, "Oh, shut up."

When the mother's in labor I check her inside to see how far she's open and when she's coming. I can tell if there's a slow birth. If they have their contractions, and the womb won't open, but a little slow, it will be a long birth.

Sometimes the mothers can't push hard, and if you help them with your hand they can push harder. There are too many people that are used to me, and they say, "Come on, Jesusita, help me. I want this baby out."

When the babies come, I like the mothers to lay down, but some of the mothers are getting new ways. Well, I don't like those; I'm not used to them. There is a book when they're on their hands and knees, but I'm not used to it. And if they're sitting, they're on the baby's head that way, so that baby have to come out up, not down like he's supposed to go. I like the old ways.

And when the lady is opening for the baby's head, I pour a little olive oil on the lady, on her perineum, by her vagina, so that part gets soft and smooth and tender, and it won't cut. So it won't tear when the baby's head come out. I massage it; I rub it so it bends more, and it doesn't rip and tear. Then I pour a little more olive oil on it and rub it some more, and the mothers feel good.

My grandmother taught me how to do that. My grandmother was a good midwife; she was number one at Trujillo. When the other midwives couldn't do it, they go and bring my grandmother, and she do it in a little while.

When the baby's head is coming out I get a white rag, and I hold it on the bottom where the baby's head is coming. I hold the head so it comes slow until it is out, and then I put the rag down below on the bed and hold the baby's head and body so it won't pop out too fast. Then, as he comes all the way out, I hold his head and hips and lay the baby down.

I clean the baby's face and eyes so the baby breathes. He's usually crying and waving his little hands, and sometimes he's scared, sometimes. Then I have to get the cord in my hand until it stops to beat. I tie it a little long, and then four fingers longer, and I tie another string. Then cut on the middle.

I wrap the new one in a blanket and give the baby to the mother for a little while. She usually is, oh, so happy and talks to her new little one. Then I take the baby back and clean the baby with olive oil and cotton. I wipe the baby all over and put drops in the eyes. And I bind the baby round with gauze. That way, when he cries, where the cord was won't pop out. Finally, I weigh the baby, and then the next day I give him a bath.

Sometimes I have to give mouth-to-mouth breathing to help that baby, sometimes. Consuelo my granddaughter helped me do it some years ago. Because sometimes she likes to help me, and once she said, "Oh, Tita, this baby's not crying; he's going to die!"

I told her, "No, shut up. If you're going to help me, shut up, and come and give mouth-to-mouth." So she did. Oh, she was proud because she makes that baby cry.

I didn't want Consuelo to scare the mother. I don't say anything to scare them. If she have a breech baby I never let her know, because they get so scared. A breech is a little hard for the mother 'cause it's a little big. First his bottom comes out and then his legs and feets. Then you have to put your left hand under the baby's chin when his head starts to come. You raise the feets a little bit, not too much, so that head will slide down. Now I take the mother with a breech baby to the hospital, but I used to deliver her.

Some fathers and mothers want to put the baby in a little tub of warm water as soon as he born. Just the last little while they do it. Oh, I like to see them do that. The babies relax, and they quit crying. They look everywhere, yes. The father have to do that; that's the way they baptize that baby. I put the baby in the father's hands, and he puts it in the water. Oh, that's pretty. That's wonderful, I love it. See, everyday you learn something, everyday. You never through learning, never. The more you live the more you learn.

Sometimes I have to get blood for special tests. The doctors bring me little bottles. So I can get that blood, and they're supposed to take it to the hospital. They have to check it from the cord and the afterbirth. I put the cord in the bottle, one big bottle and the other small.

I put a binder around the patient too. Take a long straight piece of white cloth and pin it around the lady, and then another piece to help with the bleeding. I put a binder on the baby and the patient because I'm an old-fashioned midwife. I learned that things from my grandmother. It makes the mother feel better, 'cause sometimes when she's going to turn, she's stomach is so soft that she don't feel better when she turn. Her stomach's kind of heavy and that binder holds her, and she feels better. When she have those cramps, that binder helps her, so the clots can come out. Yes, I'm an old-fashioned.

Then I fill out a birth certificate. They never used them when I started. In 1941, when I live in Trujillo, a nurse came there, and she bring me some blanks. She taught me how to make it and since then I do.

Once a doctor come from Santa Fe and asked me many questions and watched me. He's a midwife. What do you call it? An obstetrician. He wanted to know how I used the olive oil and how I held the baby. He asks me about the cord and what do I have to do with the cord when the baby come. He asks me so many questions. Other doctors come too. It makes me feel so good to have them come and watch me and talk with me. Like they trust me.

Sometimes something goes wrong, and I have to call a doctor or take that lady to the hospital. 'Cause I know, I know everything, like when a baby's not a normal baby. Sometimes the afterbirth is half born and just a little piece is stuck in there. I can go in and get it, but she might start to bleed. If that happens, they can do it better than I can. Now I take ladies to the hospital when a baby comes breech baby or too late. She's got too many help over there. I call the doctor, and I say I'm going to take this lady to the hospital, this and this and this happen to her, and they believe me. I'm so glad they believe me.

When I take my patient to the hospital I tell the doctor, "Don't give her any X-rays. Take her in there; she's this way and that way." The doctors found out; they trust me. I don't even have to talk to them; I just tell them with my hands 'cause I don't want that lady to hear what happened with her. 'Cause they get so scared if they hear.

Sometimes, though, there's nothing wrong. The mother's just a little scared, and she doesn't want to push. When she pushes hard she feels pain, and then she holds that baby. Yes, she suffers just because she's afraid.

A midwife also needs to know how to help the mother in other ways besides the birth. Some ladies want somebody with them during the labor, but some don't like nobody to stay with them but me, neither her husband. Once the husband was here, and he likes to be with her, but she never wants him with her. When she's in real labor, when the contraction goes away, she turns and tells him, "Go out! Go out, I don't want you here. Go out!" Yes, she get mad and throws him out. There are mothers who don't want their baby. Maybe that's what's wrong with her. She comes every year to me.

When I take care of ladies who don't want their baby, and when the baby's born, I wrap him and tell them, "Look at your baby."

"No," they say. "Get out of here. I don't like that baby."

When I'm in school I learn how to help these mothers. I wait for awhile and don't bother them, let them alone, and they change; they calm down and after a while they say, "Bring me my baby, I want to see it." You see, sometimes it's hard to be a mother.

Some mothers have too many troubles. I have one, when she was sixteen years old somebody gets her, puts her in a car, five boys, and they rape her. It's so hard on her she have to go to the state mental hospital, and she's like retarded. Her people treat her bad too.

Later she has lots of babies. Once the man that was living with her came here, and he said, "Here she is. She's going to have a baby; I have to go back home, and I don't know when I'm coming for her."

After her baby's born I make her take a bath 'cause she's real dirty, and I give her clean clothes and get some clothes too, to wrap that baby. Poor mother and poor baby.

I tell her to get some help from the clinic, so she'll not have no more babies. She says, "No Jesusita, don't make me do anything. I'm scared. You have to go with me." So I have to go with her, and the doctor helps her. And, you know what? I have to pay the taxi to send her home after her baby came. The man never cared, no. He never pays me either.

I used to help with adoptions, years ago. Girls would come from the university, young ladies who were pregnant and alone. They didn't want to keep their babies, 'cause they were too scared. And I give their babies away, to good people. 'Cause I know everybody, and they always ask me for babies. Oh, some of them are grown now. The new parents are so glad they don't know what to do with it. They say, "Thanks, Jesusita, thanks." They don't know what to say, they're so happy. 'Cause some ladies don't have babies, never. They like them good, like they were their own babies.

Sometimes when babies were born, the baby died, and then the mothers, oh, they feel so bad. I deliver triplets once. They were five months along and were all dead. The mother felt so bad, she cries a lot. She was so sorry for her little babies. She felt so sorry, even though she had ten others at home.

I try to help the mothers when their babies die, just tell them that those things happen and try to make them happy. Well, not happy, but feel better. It's hard. It's hard to make them feel good. Not so good, but to understand.

Yes, there's much sadness. Juanita, my cousin, had her baby boy. She never before have a baby boy. She's got four girls, and she never had a baby boy until last year and that baby was dead. A doctor delivered the boy, and I had delivered the girls. See, it sometimes happen, even with a doctor. It seems there is much sadness no matter what.

I know how people can hurt. That's part the reason I don't charge too much. They ask me the other day, on the clinic, "Why don't you charge one hundred dollars? Everything is going high; why don't you, Jesusita?" Because I don't want to, and I work for my own. I'm my own boss; that's why they don't make me. I want to help the people; they need help. I know they have money, some of them, they can give one hundred dollars for their time, but I don't want to do that. I feel better to charge fifty.

Sometimes somebody comes in here, and they're crying and saying, "Jesusita, I need you, but I don't have any money. I'm going to have a baby, and I don't have any money."

So I tell them, "OK, just come in. You can have your baby here, and you don't have to pay me if you don't have any money." And when they go home, in a month or two, they come and bring my money.

It's hard to be good midwife sometimes. It's not easy, no.

I had a neighbor who used to live in the green house near me. She said, she told me one night, "Anybody can be a midwife, that's easy."

And I told her, "Why didn't you do it?"

She said that 'cause one of her sisters have a baby. After the baby's born, the father said, "How much do I owe you, Jesusita?"

And I told him, "Twenty-five dollars." I charge twenty-five dollars at that time.

My neighbor heard that and said, "Well, anybody can be a midwife, that's too much."

I told her, "No, not everybody. You'll find out some day." And she did, she find out.

Later my neighbor moved to a different street, near her girl. Her girl was having a baby, and I was called. Her girl was very bad. My neighbor said, "What's the matter with Rose Ann?"

And I told her, "She's very sick, very, very sick."

My neighbor said, "Do you think you can do it?"

I said, "I think so."

She then said, "Can I stay here?"

"No, you can't stay." You see, it was too hard. Rose Ann had a very hard time.

They could hear Rose Ann cry with so much pain, but after a long time I deliver her baby, and the baby's OK and Rose Ann is OK too. I clean the baby and everything and let my neighbor in.

She say, "No, not everybody can be a midwife. Thanks, Jesusita." Yes, she found out. Maybe a year had gone by, and then she know this.

I help peoples in lots of ways. I get so many calls, and people come so much to my door. Sometimes they come just to see how I am, but most of the time they want to know something; what is good for this, for that, for that. They come not just for babies. Sometimes they come for the stomach, sometimes for a womb. Sometimes, if they feel a pain, and it's the womb hurting them, I know how to fix it.

Lots people come to know if they should go to a doctor or to the hospital. Not long ago my friend Anita hurts a finger, and it's bleeding, and she come to me. She wants to know if she should show it to a doctor. I say, "Yes" and it's infected, so she needs to stay in the hospital, and they operate on her finger.

Once she fell down in her house. Oh, she was bleeding a lot from her head. So her son Antonio came crying, "Tita, come on. My mother is dying, my mother is bleeding. She fell down and hit her head on the corner, and she open her head." So I went there and get towels and wet them in cold water and put them around the head to try to stop that bleeding until the taxi come and get her to the hospital.

She calls me first before she goes to the hospital. That's the way they do; everybody calls me first. I can help them just a little, sometimes I can help them OK, but sometimes I have to send them to the hospital.

Two ladies came today. One is pregnant with her third. She came and told me that she has a white discharge, and I told her, "You better go and see the doctor. I can't do that." So she goes.

Sometimes the woman go to the doctor and ask them if they are pregnant. They are only one or two months. The doctor checks them and says, "No, I don't think so."

So they come back to me, and they say, "Jesusita, I came to see you, I think I'm pregnant." So I check them, and I can tell them when they are one month. Two is easy.

And I can tell them when it's a tumor. Sometimes they're going to the doctor and going to the doctor and go and say, "I don't know what's the matter with me; I have a hard pain," but the doctor can't say.

So they come to me, and I check them, and I call the doctor that is taking care of them, and I tell him, "Did you know what's the matter with this? This is your patient, and she came to see me."

The doctor says, "No."

I say, "I know, she's going back to you and give her some X-rays. She's got a tumor." And they take my word, the doctors.

From Denver they come. From California came one not long ago. I used to know her, and she said, "I don't know what's the matter with the doctor. He don't do me anything.

I'm going to see him every week or every two days." You know what, she's got a tumor as big as a hand. I don't know how the doctors don't know that. After I found out she went and had her operation in Santa Fe.

One lady came to me and said, "Tita, what's the matter with me. I'm always dripping, dripping." And I told her, "You go and tell the doctor about that." So he gave her a hysterectomy. He was afraid she had some cancer 'cause that dripping came from inside.

The other day I have one. Oh, she was so sick, so sick she can hardly stand. She have a pain in her right side. The family calls me 'cause she can't get up.

I go and examine that girl, and it's a tube baby, and this was the second baby she looses. She had a miscarriage with her first. She was, oh, so anxious to have one OK and is crying and feeling so bad.

I call the obstetrician right away and tell him I have a girl like this, and he says, "Tell her to come right over."

He operate on her that night, and it was a tube baby like I said.

Then he calls me and tells me, "Jesusita, how did you know this?"

I tell him, "I don't know, I just use my hands, no instruments, and my hands can tell."

I'm sorry for that girl but glad for her too. Before there were the doctors, there was nothing we could do for a lady with a tube baby. She would just die, that's all, but it's not like that now. Now she can live.

I have another girl who called for me, not so many years ago. It was before she was married. She was very, very sick.

She said to her father, "I want Jesusita to see me because I'm going to die today, Daddy." The doctor didn't know what was the matter with her, she's just so sick.

So I went there, and I told her, "Do you want me to examine you? You're very sick down there, but maybe I shouldn't touch you 'cause you're still a virgin."

And she told me, "Go ahead and do it; the doctors do anything they want to with me."

So I examine her. Do you know what's the matter? A big

ımor in her womb. And I tell her father and her mother, and I tell them to take her to Santa Fe because that tumor is going to bust, and if it busts she will die.

But her daddy says, "No, I know she's not going to die because you know what's the matter with her? She's pregnant, that's why she is bleeding and swelling. She's a bad girl, that's why."

The girl says, "No, no Daddy. I'm not pregnant, I'm sick. I never do nothing bad."

I say, "That's true, she did nothing to be ashamed of, she is sick."

So her mother and aunt take her to Santa Fe, and I call the doctor and say, "It's an emergency." So they operate right away, and the girl lives and is well and happy.

She's married and in Colorado now, and everytime she comes to see her mother, she comes to see me. She never forgets, and her mother says, "If it wasn't for you my daughter would be dead."

I tell her, "No, it's God. God do everything for me." And that's how I feel. God helps me, and when I touch people they feel better 'cause they trust me. You see, I just use my hands and my mind, my hands and my mind and God.

Sometimes ladies come to me who have been hurt bad. Once I treated a girl who was raped. She was so swollen she could hardly walk. Two boys do it. Oh, she cried and cried, because her boyfriend was in the army, and she was waiting for him to get married with him. She cried, and she said, "Oh, he isn't going to love me anymore. He isn't." But he did. She called him, and he came to see her, and he cried too. They both feel so bad.

Sometimes I help a man. They maybe twist a foot, a wrist, or his neck, something. But I don't like to do that, no, but I do it, sometimes I do it. And I fix one man who had a wound in his stomach that wouldn't heal. I fix some herbs and put it on and before long, it's better.

And sometimes I help the children. I help them with the *empacho.* I don't know if there's English for it; I don't think so. The kids get it when they eat or chew or swallow something bad for them, and it's stuck in there. Maybe they eat too much cold lunch or too much potato chips with coke, so I have to rub the stomach and back to put it down, and I pull the skin up and clack it, so it's loose in there. I learn this from my grandma long ago.

I know what's good for a fever besides aspirin. Rubbing alcohol on the body and *azafrán*, if you make a tea. It's a flower, a red thing, and you make a tea and give it to them. We used to do that in Trujillo. We used to plant too many azafrán. I can't hardly find the seed now, it's a little white weed.

There are others. The *escoba de la víbora*, that's snakeweed; it's for ulcers. Make tea and drink it, and *mastranzo* just the same, for the same thing. And *romerillo* is for hemorrhages. There are so many that I can't remember. But I remember some of them. They used them when people were sick when I was little, and sometimes now.

This mastranzo is good for those little things that grow in the vagina, the yeast infection. Use mastranzo and *añil del muerto*. Just boil it, make tea, and put them in a douche bag and douche with it. And drink some. I have some; yes, everybody brings me herbs.

And *immortal* is good for the heart. And if somebody was just weak, a baby was sickly and weak, we give *manzanilla*, chamomile, to drink. It's good for mothers too, cleans it out, when they have those cramps, afterbirth pain. And we give her *pazote* to drink; sweet basil is pazote. There were lots of things, lots of herbs to help with.

My grandmother showed me how to use these things. When I was little. She learned them from her mother. Everybody knew them back then, and they teach each other. Yes, I know many things now. I'm partera, a midwife, and some people say I'm médica. I'm médica, the healer.

Yes, there is so many things to remember, so many things to happen. Now I have good times sometimes and sadness sometimes, too many sadness sometimes.

Ernesto is divorced, about eight years. I don't know why; I don't know why. And my girl, Dolores, has trouble too. She works at the State Hospital with the children's unit now. I've got good children, but sometimes have such troubles.

It's hard for me. My face don't show it, but my heart.

'Cause everybody tell me, "Oh, you look so glad and you feel healthy." Yes, I'm healthy, thanks to God. But I feel so sad for my children.

And I have my little troubles with my boy and my granddaughters and my grandsons. Sometimes they don't want to do what I tell them to do. Sometimes my grandchildren are invited to parties, parties that are no good. I worry about them and can't go away from my troubles.

My son used to play in a band and sing at the radio station in Albuquerque. I hear him on the radio here. I saw him on television every Saturday. He doesn't anymore, and sometimes he's sad, but he lives in the house next to mine, and I help him.

He's a good son with me. He says to me all the time, "I don't want to die after you, I want to die before you die. 'Cause I'm going to miss you a lot. I don't know what I'm going to do without you." Yes, I have good children and good grandchildren.

I have other troubles besides my worries about my family. You know what happened the other day? A Mexican lady is going to have a baby, and somebody said, "Where?"

And the lady answered, "With Jesusita."

"No," that person said, "She can't do it. Jesusita is pretty near to the end of the line." I don't know why they say that. I hurt and don't know why.

Lots of times I also have trouble with my house. I had to call the man, the plumber, again a few days ago. And it cost me $20.85. And I always have trouble with that line, always. Sometimes the pipe busts outside, and they are digging and digging and digging. I'm so sick and tired of those lines.

Some of my problems come from my boarders. I started taking in outpatients from the mental hospital about ten years ago. You know why I have to put a boarding house? Because the women were using those birth control. But I don't blame the ladies for using the birth control, I would have when I was young. But I don't have enough babies to make my living with such few ladies, so I have to see what else I can do. I couldn't go back to work on the factory or somewhere else because I was sixty years old. So I take the outpatients. I put four of them in the room I used to use for mothers and babies, back when I had many at the same time.

Now I'm my own boss again, taking care of those four patients. And they're good to me; they're good patients. Oh, sometimes, you know, they get a little strange, but that's the way they are. I notice that it depends on the weather. One of them can't talk and can't hear. But I write to him, and he writes me back. He's got a good English.

I have to do everything for the patients. I cook for them and wash for them. I clean their room and check on them to be sure they're OK. They're always coming and going in my house, and I have to watch them. I got some of the patients who used to drink, and I don't let them drink and then they feel better. Oh no, I don't let them drink.

When they get their checks, if I notice they drink something, I tell them, "Don't you ever do that again." I say, "I'm going to call the police and send you to sleep there." So they quit.

And if somebody, some other patient, comes here and asks them to go out with them to drink, I tell my patients, "No, you're not supposed to do that." Then I say to the other person, "No sir, you go by yourself."

He says, "They let me."

I say, "Well, if they let you, I don't care, but my patients ain't going to drink." Yes, they are not going to drink; I don't let them.

I also have to give my patients their medicine. Three patients takes two pills three times a day, another takes one in the day and two at night. I can give shots too. I used to have one with sugar diabetes, and I have to give him a shot everyday. Yeah, I learned to do that 'cause I have my pin, my home nursing pin. I do many things for the patients, and I'm not lying; I'm telling the truth. I'm working hard, working so hard.

Even though I have to watch the patients, most of the time I sleep good at night, if I don't have a lady here. My room is close to the patients, and sometimes I hear them, though. Then I get up and get my flashlight and go in there. Sometimes one of them is just drinking water.

You know, I know so many mothers of my patients. They come from far away and talk with me, and they like to meet me. They feel so bad their sons had to be in the hospital, and they want to see where they live, now their sons are out.

The caseworker from Santa Fe in charge of my boarders came not long ago. He wasn't the regular one and was so hateful. He said that I have to paint the boarders' room. I know that I have to paint it; he don't have to tell me, but some people think you don't do these things 'cause you don't want to. No, sometimes you can't. You just don't have enough money.

I have life insurance, and I ask my insurance for a little money to fix my house and paint it and everything. You know how much they send me? Twelve dollars, just twelve dollars, so I tell him, "I don't want that check, send it back." That's not even enough for a gallon of paint, and I need three gallons for that room.

You know what else they say when they come from Santa Fe to inspect. They want me to have some magazines for the patients. You know why I don't have any papers there? Because one of them start a fire, twice. So the inspectors don't know anything how to take care of these people. They come and tell me this and that and that and that, and they don't even know how to take care of them.

They say, "Put in another window, and make a manual, and put the hour and the date you give them a fire alarm."

You know, I have a whistle, but the patients don't care about it. When I get in there and whistle they don't say anything, no. I have to tell them, "Go out! Learn how to go out. Learn how to run from the fire." No, they don't know.

With two boarders you don't have to have a license. But I don't have enough money with two, no. I have to have four. I have to take care of the outpatients, my grandchildren, and everybody. Yesterday I get so tired. Oh, when I was washing the floor in there, oh, I can hardly breathe, I was so tired. Sometimes when I get so tired when I'm taking care of the patients, I say, "Maybe I take care of them this year, but maybe if I get tired and tired, I have to quit doing that." I've been taking care of these people ten years.

Many people, many ladies that have taken care of these people, they quit. They get tired and sick. So they decide to put the patients away, but if you quit working, you don't have any help, no.

I keep trying to think of what to do. They said the other day that there is a program to help the old people with the utilities, and I'm going to try it, maybe tomorrow. I'm going to *Sierras y Llanos*. There is where you fill a paper and tell how much you make. I'm going to try, 'cause worrying like this is so hard for the last of your life. I never thought that I have to work this hard when I'm getting old. No, I never think of it, never.

Sometimes I don't get much sleep for many nights. A while ago I was up all night for a lady and then up the next night with another, helping them with their babies. Then I get a good night's sleep and have to get up at six in the morning and start washing. I washed all day and then another lady came that night for her baby. I get too tired, doing all that.

Lots of the time I have so many clothes to wash. The patients' and my grandchildren's and mine, all in my wringer washer and hang outside. Lots of time I have three days of washing to do.

Not long ago I went to my cousin's for dinner 'cause my nephew; they baptize my nephew's baby, and he come and invite me for dinner. So I went and have dinner with them, but I almost never go anywhere 'cause I want to be sure to be here for my ladies, in case they call me. But I went then and had dinner, but as soon as I got in I have to work.

People say to sit and watch TV to rest, but when I sit down to watch TV, I go to sleep. I'm tired, that's why. Somebody told me, "Maybe you're sick."

I say, "No, I'm not sick; I'm tired."

Sometimes when nobody comes to visit me, I feel a long day, and I'm always falling asleep. And when everybody comes to visit, I feel so happy. See, that's what makes me feel good, the people. Somebody come here and talk me that and that, and others come and give me a good time. Yes, maybe God will help us all someday.

Now I'm old. Most of the time I'm too busy to think, but,

sometimes, when I'm alone and it's quiet late at night, I sit in my rocking chair and I think and I remember. I remember all those that are gone, my mother, father, grandparents, the ranch with too many good things, good things to remember. But I also think of troubles. Worries for my kids and grandkids, and think of all the poor ladies and babies I take care of. I think of the good things we had and the hard times we had. I think of the hard times for too many people in Trujillo and here.

I think of why people are so poor, so many poor ladies all along. I think that there's no more rain, that there's not too many jobs, and I think that people don't have their land and that people are unhappy and drink. I think of single mothers who are afraid to ask their parents for money, and I think of ladies whose husbands don't want to work or they're getting drunk all the time, and that's why they don't have money. Some of those men don't care; they don't even come for their ladies.

That's the people that need the welfare. They really need it, but sometimes welfare don't want to help her 'cause I know too many people like that. Many people bring me clothes, and I give to ones I know need it. These are the ones that need help sometimes, help so they won't have more and more babies.

I think some men don't treat their ladies too good. Sometimes they make me cry in front of the ladies 'cause I feel sad for them, I feel sorry for them. A good thing that I don't have a husband, if that's the way that he was going to treat me, no thanks.

But sometimes it's good not to have a husband and sometimes it's hard. You know why? It's hard because when you need something you have to go on your own and ask for it and sometimes you get it, sometimes you don't. Like if you need money, to borrow money from somewhere, the bank or finance, and they don't let you have it. Sometimes, then, I feel it's better for me to be dead. I come home and cry sometimes, and, you know, in a little while somebody comes and says, "I'm going to have my baby."

"Oh, Lord," I say, "Thank you. You have to help me."

That's all I keep saying all the time. It's hard to live, but you make it one way or another; you make it and get strong.

I heard a few mornings ago that this president is going to take away the welfare from the people. I don't know how, too many people need that, needs help. There are too many mothers that have too many kids, and they don't have no work. They need the help; they need the welfare, otherwise they would be hungry.

President Kennedy was a good man. He was trying to straighten up everything and to see that the people could live and don't be in war. He try to help everybody, poor people too. When President Kennedy died everybody cries. And I watch that, I was delivering a baby when he died, and I saw everything on television. They named that baby John, and I watch until they bury the president, and I cried for him. I feel so sorry for him, and everybody cries for him. I keep his picture on my wall 'cause he was important to us; he tried to help.

You know, I think of all the troubles my ladies have with their families, and I think I'm glad they have those birth control now. Even if fewer mothers come to me. Yes, the Lord knows that people have to use birth control. He knows they're poor; they can't support big family. I don't believe He gets mad. Oh no, 'cause I always pray and believe on Him, and the Lord thinks, "No, they're not hurting nobody."

I also sit and think of my own trouble when I'm young, and I think if I was young I would use the birth control pills, but in those years, when I was young, nothing. You didn't know nothing about this, nothing. When you learn, it's too late. Lots of us learn too late.

I think of the other troubles people have now. People drink more than they used to; I don't know why, everybody. Women, girls, boys, and men. Oh, that's terrible. They used to drink for fun once in a year, but now, every day, every day.

I don't like to drink. Oh, sometimes I like to drink peach brandy, a little because it's sweet. I don't like sour drinks. Not beer, I don't like beer. I don't like wine, just a little peach brandy, that's all, and just once in a while.

When kids drink they do every wrong things, 'cause

they're drinking and using every kind of drugs. They get wild. They don't know what they're doing, and driving, driving fast and getting a wreck. Get hurt and everything, or killed. They don't care; they don't care for their lives, no. Some die, and there's so much sadness. It's a worry to have children now, such a worry.

Sometimes I get real scared. When my grandchildrens were small they always stay with me, and they still are with me now, but, you know, they go out, and it scares me. It scares me 'cause you know how drugs and everything is now, getting drunk and using this and using that and the fights and everything.

I think Las Vegas was a better place to live when I first came, 'cause of the kids. Kids used to obey, but now, no, no, no. It's different now. Now they get in trouble all the time, getting drunk and doing too many things. It's hard for parents here because they worry, and there's more, more people. But I like it before, more peaceful with less people.

And it's hard to talk alone and be private now. Years ago they don't let us kids stay there and listen to everything the grownups say, no. With their eyes they tell you to go. If you don't go, you get it when the company go out to their homes.

Now kids don't pay no attention to your eyes. It's hard to make them understand. I don't know why. Once I asked a doctor about this, about these modern kids who don't mind. You know what he told me?

"Don't you get mad if I tell you," he said.

"No, I won't. I'm asking you why."

"Because they are drinking milk instead of nursing when they're babies. That's why, that's one of the things. That's why," he answered me.

And I believe that. But I think it's also harder now for kids to grow. They don't know so much what to do with themselves. Things have changed a lot, and there's no more land.

Back then, when they built the Storrie Lake, when my daddy worked there and my mama died, there was lots of work for all to do. They moved the dirt with a team of horses, plows, shovels, picks, and bars. Now they can't do that; everything is made by machines. And not many people have jobs, just a little, some people that can drive a tractor or other kind of machine. So, there's not much work for the kids when they grow.

Things have changed for girls now, too, in good ways some. They are free to do what they want to. Because you had to obey your parents years ago. The parents don't let you go away from home or go to school then, and the girls feel bad.

Now they let the girls do things like that. If the family don't let them, the girls will go anyway. They say to their parents, "I go, and I have to go. I have to do something and learn something. So you have to keep quiet and that's all."

I have a niece in California who graduated from college, and she's going to be a doctor. She can talk three languages. If I have the chance to do what she's doing now, when I was young, I do it. But they didn't give me any chance. I don't know why. Maybe they could not afford it or what, but I know they could 'cause they had money. They didn't believe on that things then. That's why. Now they do this, and they let them go. Yes, my niece is going to do it. Her father told me, "She is just like you."

And I have another one that I baptized, and her mother said, "Oh, she's just like you. She likes to work, and if she needs wood she don't bother nobody, she gets the truck and goes and gets some wood." So I feel so proud.

I have 11,924 babies I deliver and from the babies I deliver, teachers, nurses, and musician. One is my godson and he is a doctor. When he graduates from medical school they come and see me, and I'm, oh, so proud. I feel happy when I know what the kids are doing. I like those babies like if they were my own. I don't know why, but I do. I don't know how to explain to you how I feel about it, but I feel so proud. And their parents say, "They are just like you. 'Cause you are always working and doing this and that." So I feel so proud.

But I would change everything if I could go back again to my ranch. Sometimes when I go there I don't want to come back. I feel so happy, so happy and healthy. That wind and sun makes me feel good. I think because I was raised there. It's when I have those troubles, that's when I feel like going back to Trujillo, to stay there and cry and rest and be by myself. Back there where there aren't problems, and I can rest and nobody with me.

I don't blame the old people that don't want to move. They want to stay where they belong, but I have to stay here and work. 'Cause I have to take care of people. Yes, I love my ranch, but I love my people. I have to stay here with my people.

ILLUSTRATIONS

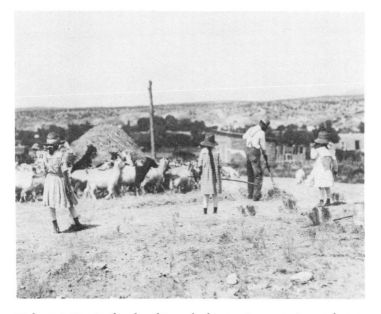

Girls assisting in the threshing of wheat using goats in northeastern New Mexico at the time of Jesusita's childhood. (*Courtesy of Museum of New Mexico.*)

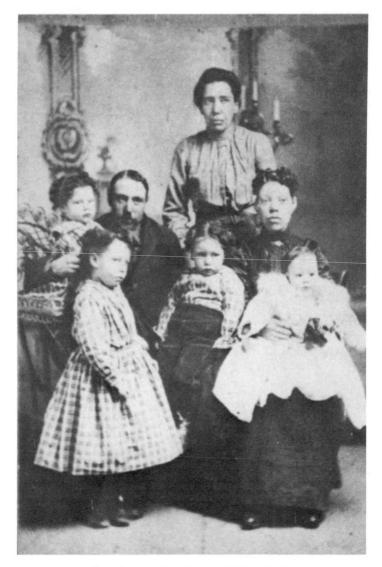

Jesusita's grandmother and family, ca. 1905. *Clockwise from top*: Jesusita's paternal grandmother Dolores Córdova Gallegos, Dolores's niece Emilia Aragón, Dolores's nephew José Manuel Aragón, and their children.

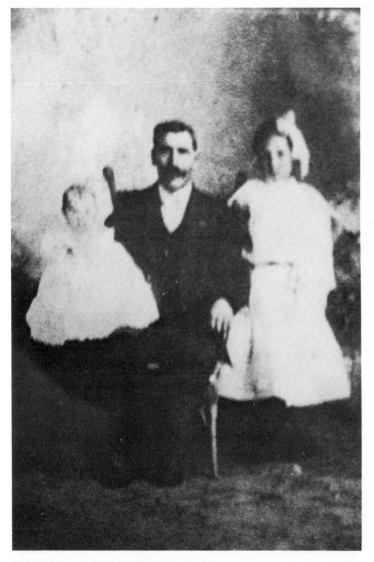

Jesusita as a baby in 1908. *Left to right*: Jesusita, Jesusita's grandfather Trinidad Gallegos, Jesusita's aunt Filomena.

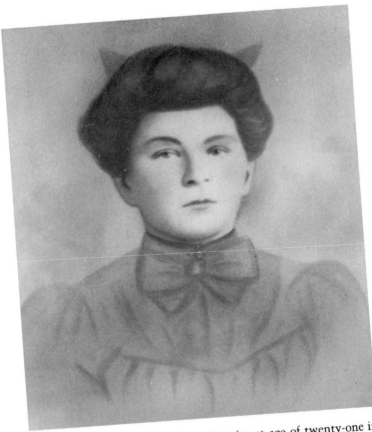

Jesusita's mother, Antonia Otero Aragón, at age of twenty-one in 1906.

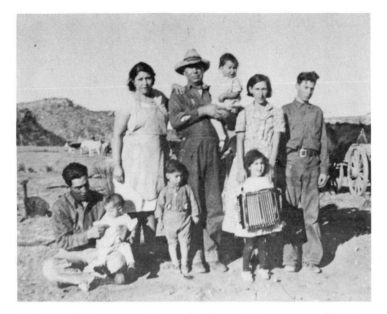

Jesusita's father, stepmother, and various relatives on ranch in Trujillo, ca. 1938. Jesusita's father is in the middle and her stepmother is second from the right.

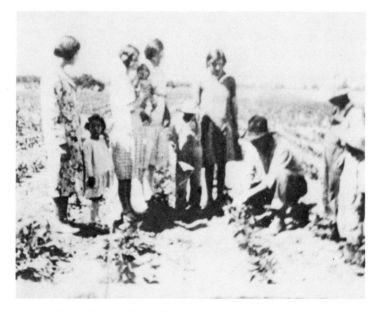

Jesusita's family in a bean field on the ranch in Trujillo, ca. 1926. *Left to right:* Jesusita's friend Beatrice Crespín with her niece; Jesusita at age eighteen holding her baby half sister Josie; Jesusita's sister Ramona; a half brother; Jesusita's sister Soledad; Jesusita's father, Thomas Aragón; two half brothers.

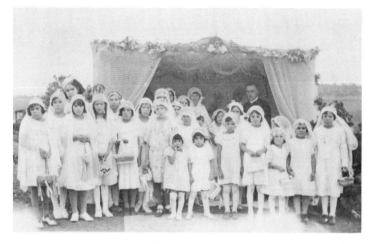

Niñas de Maria at Corpus Christi celebration in front of an outdoor altar, May 27, 1937.

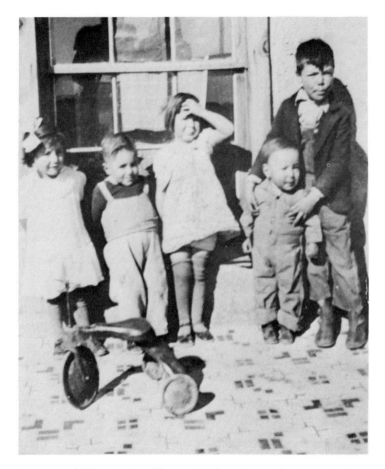

Jesusita's children in Trujillo, ca. 1939. *Left to right*: Antonia Tru-jillo, a cousin who weighed three pounds at birth; Pete Trujillo, also a cousin; Dolores, Jesusita's daughter; Ben, Jesusita's nephew; Ernesto, Jesusita's son.

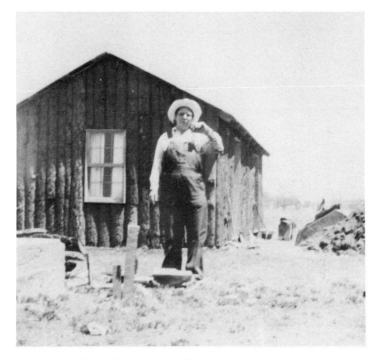

Jesusita building her house and maternity center in Las Vegas, 1953.

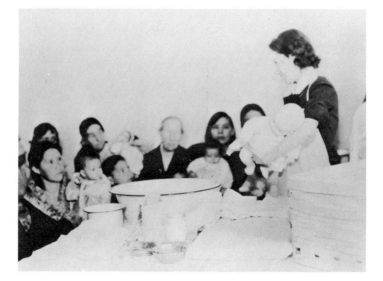

Village home hygiene class taught by public health nurses, 1937. *Far left,* midwife Cipriana Sena; *above second from left,* midwife Josefita Gallegos; *far right,* nurse trainee Marie Casias holding doll.

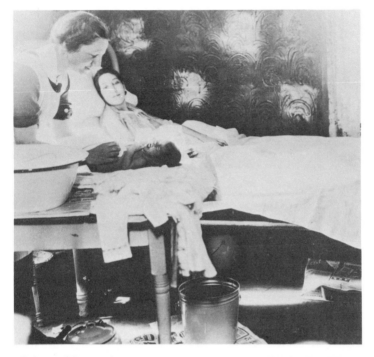

Edith Rackley making home visit to new mother in Las Vegas, 1937.

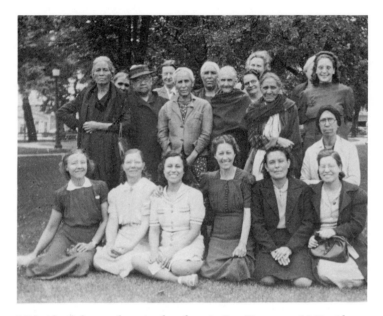

Midwife club members in the plaza in Las Vegas, ca. 1941. *Above third from left,* Carmelita Ardones; *fourth from left,* Dr. Nancy Campbell; *below left,* Olive Nicklin; *second from left,* Jesusita Aragón; *far right,* Aurelia Gutiérrez.

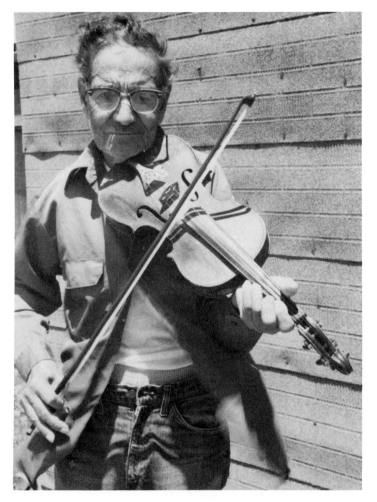

Gregorio Parson, longtime neighbor of Jesusita and musician for village festivals and dances, 1978. Photograph by the author.

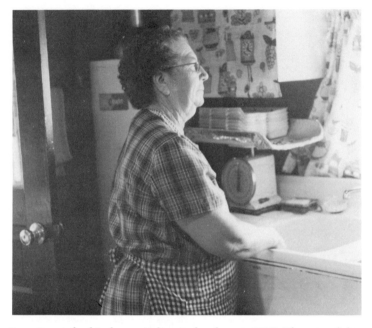

Jesusita at the kitchen window in her home, 1978. Photograph by the author.

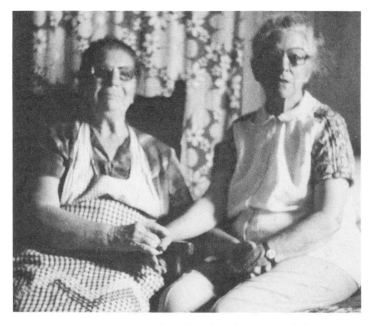

Jesusita Aragón and retired public health nurse Edith Rackley, 1977. Photograph by the author.

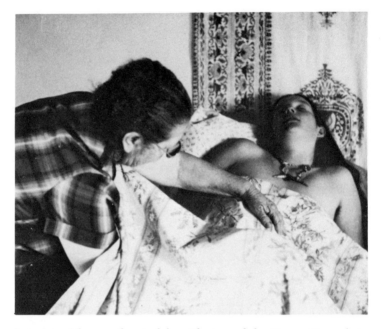

Jesusita with a mother in labor. Photograph by Steven Oppenheimer.

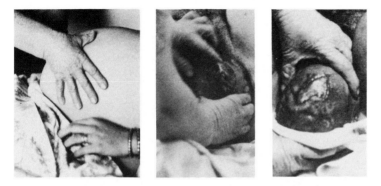

Left: Jesusita's hands on the mother's stomach during labor. Photograph by Steven Oppenheimer. *Center*: Massaging the perineum with olive oil to prevent tearing. Photograph by the author. *Right*: Supporting the infant's head in a faceup position. Photograph by the author.

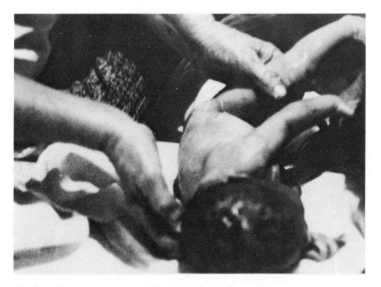

Birth in faceup position. Photograph by the author.

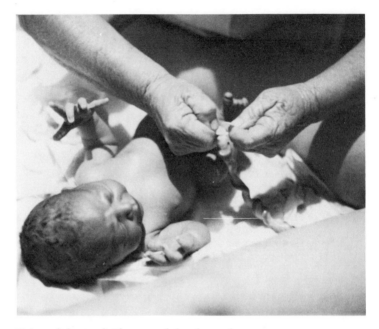

Tying of the cord. Photograph by the author.

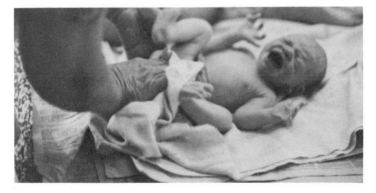

Cleaning the infant immediately following birth. Photograph by
Paul Pearlman.

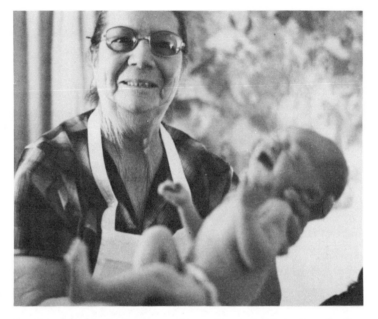

Jesusita showing the infant to the mother and father seconds after birth. Photograph by Steven Oppenheimer.

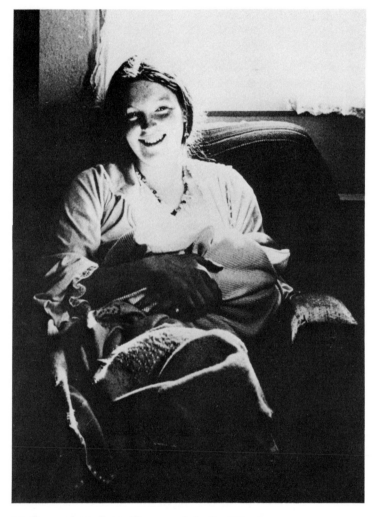

Mother and newborn. Photograph by Paul Pearlman.

APPENDICES

1. Networks

THERE WERE UNIQUE medical needs in northeastern New
Mexico during the end of the nineteenth century and the
early part of the twentieth century. The area at that time
was experiencing poverty, the breakdown of the existing
culture, a period of droughts, and isolation from the dominant Anglo medical care system that had developed and was
serving most of the rest of the country.

These conditions created extensive health care needs, including a need for preventive and therapeutic medical care,
improved nutrition, and maternity and infant care. A number of these medical needs were responded to for an extended period of time by cooperative networks of primarily
female health care givers. This was true in the early period,
during the time of the curanderas and parteras, when a majority of the healers were female,[1] and later, after the introduction of Anglo medical care.[2]

Because of the importance of the town of Las Vegas to the
region, some medical doctors had arrived relatively early,
and, by 1881, the Las Vegas Medical Society, with eight en-
rolled members, was formed.[3] The majority of the doctors
did not go out to the villages, however, and so the people in
the surrounding areas did not receive such medical care.[4]

Several women's groups developed the two hospitals in
the area. In 1883 the Ladies' Relief Society banded together
"to relieve the sick and needy," as it was stated in the local

newspaper at that time, and, under the leadership of Mrs. L. N. Higgins, they opened a small hospital in 1888. This eventually developed into the Las Vegas Hospital which was incorporated in 1911.[5]

In 1895 the Sisters of Charity, located in Leavenworth, Kansas, decided to establish a hospital in Las Vegas for tubercular patients. It opened in January, 1897, and eventually became St. Anthony's hospital in Las Vegas.[6] In addition, there were women among the early private physicians in the area. Dr. Mary Lou Hickman was the first medical doctor with a private practice in Las Vegas who then began to assist with the public health clinic, and Dr. M. L. Christie, a black woman osteopath who came to Las Vegas in the 1920s, had an extensive practice in all of Las Vegas and was well respected in the area.

As a result of Presbyterian medical outreach women doctors also came and set up clinics in the general region. Dr. Sarah Bowen was a pioneer in such care. She set up a clinic in Dixon, New Mexico, in 1934, and school teachers from throughout the area, including San Miguel County, brought people to her clinic. The clinic was developed in 1940 into Embudo Hospital and was used as a base for other clinics that Dr. Bowen started in Chamisa, Holman, Chacón, and Truchas. A similar medical outreach during a later period of time helped Dr. Edith Millican to start in 1957 the Mora Valley Clinic in a rural area not far from Las Vegas.

Yet, despite the availability of these resources, many people in the rural areas of San Miguel County did not get needed help from the early hospitals and physicians.[7] Transportation problems, economics, and cultural differences all contributed to this lack of care, and large parts of the county continued with its earlier forms of medical care. Edith Rackley, one of the first public health nurses in the area, stated that when she first began working in San Miguel County in 1936, 95 percent of all the births in the county were attended by midwives. She also commented that, in spite of the midwives' efforts, the county had one of the highest infant mortality rates in the country.

Many factors contributed to the infant mortality rate at

that time. One of the factors was malnutrition. During extensive personal interviews, Edith Rackley stated:

There were a lot of sad things for everybody to deal with. There were many babies and mothers lost where malnutrition was a factor. It often happened because they just couldn't get food because of the droughts and general poverty and because the diet had been changed so that many just weren't getting the nutrition they needed. The mothers were just overworked and underfed.

The few babies who were not able to be nursed had a hard time, a very hard time, and many of these babies had to be on formulas just because of the mother's run down condition, because the mothers were too weak to supply an adequate diet for the infant. But the formula costs a lot of money, and they had no way to refrigerate it.

I remember one time I went to a home and told a mother how to set up the formula, and then I came back. She lived in a tiny, little old house with just one little north window, and she had found a bucket that would hold the jar that she made and kept the formula in. She had the bucket with water in it hanging in the dark window with the bottle in it and a rag over it. That's how she kept it cool. But that poor mother died, and she had cared so much to help her baby.

Throughout this period, the lay midwives continued to serve their people. Jesusita tells that when she moved to Las Vegas in 1952, about sixty-five midwives were still working in the town. Of these midwives, Señora Carmen Cidio, Señora Aurelia Gutiérrez, and Señora Gabrielita Lucero are still alive but in retirement. Dr. Edith Millican also speaks of the continued importance of the midwives and states that when the Mora Valley Clinic was started in 1957, about ten midwives were still practicing in the valley and getting back up services from the hospital in Dixon.

Edith Rackley spoke of the importance of the midwives to the villages and said:

When I came in 1936 the midwives were very important people in their villages, and they helped with many other things besides births. Lots of places they were called médicas. We might ask for the partera, the midwife, when we went into a village, and in the conversation the word médica would come out. The médica served all the medical needs and, often, whatever ailment they had, they went to the midwife. The midwives often dispensed herbs for different complaints and also played the part of a counselor to the villagers.

The midwife was the only type of leader in a village community except for the men who were politically inclined, and, of course, except for the religious leaders. People would go to the midwife because there was no other woman leader. It was the only profession open for women, unless they could go to town and be a teacher. So, the midwife was a very special person, especially for the other women.[8]

For the past forty years public health programs have supplemented and upgraded the care given by these midwives and have performed important roles in the health care delivery system of this area. These programs have met a variety of medical needs for people unable to afford private physicians.

Public health was first introduced into San Miguel County in 1936 as a demonstration unit in maternal and child care, funded by the United States Children's Bureau.[9] Since then it has developed extensive programs giving a variety of services and is a model of what such departments can do.

Most of the public health workers in San Miguel County have been women. Edith Rackley stated that when she became supervising nurse in 1938 the staff of twelve were all women. A photo taken in 1939 of the persons employed by the San Miguel County Health Department shows that eleven of the thirteen employees were women.[10]

Edith Rackley remembered the means of reaching people when public health first came into the area:

We were to develop a generalized health program for families, and in order to start reaching the people we were to set up general health clinics in the schools. The county was divided up, and I was given the eastern part of the county. I had sixty-six schools; seven of them I couldn't reach by car. They were, in most cases, just one little adobe room, often times separate from the house, and maybe just the children that lived in that immediate vicinity went to that school.

To set up the clinics we made denim curtains and had them on hooks. We took out wires which we'd hang across and divide the room and put the curtains on. The room we'd use was in a school, a vacant house, or even once an empty barn, and then we'd carry in our heavy boxes of equipment. We tried to teach people through classes. We called them home hygiene classes, and it was in one of these classes, out in the area of Trujillo, that I met Jesusita.

We also set up classes in which midwives were taught. Those women satisfactorily completing them could be certified to practice midwifery. By that time we had a nurse-midwife assigned to our service who did nothing but work with the midwives. She would conduct the classes and teach them. They were taught to have a bag fully equipped for home delivery with things clean, boiled, ironed, and wrapped. These were taught the importance of cleanliness and the technical procedure of delivery. They were also taught the danger signals, to recognize them early, and they were given telephone numbers to call to get help.

Later the nurse-midwife service was not continued, but the field nurses did continue to work with the midwives. The midwives were organized into a club, and they would come once a month into the Health Department, and someone of us would be there to meet with them. We also gave them fresh, sterile supplies.

In addition, we did prenatal exams and gave back up services. One night, long ago, the physician called me and said, "We've had a call from a midwife to go out." So, I went with her, and we got out there; the woman had been in labor a long time. We had lamps to hold, and the doctor found that this woman had twins, and one was in the way of the other, and they were in trouble. So she had to put on her big gloves and go in the mother and get one of those babies and straighten her out. We had two of the darlingest, little tiny girls you ever saw. They were round and plump, just tiny.

It was late at night, and we fixed them little beds. We padded a box and heated old irons and bricks and things for warmth since they didn't have hot water bottles, and so we got those babies all fixed up. And then I went back and visited them a number of times, and they were fine.

Infant death statistics in New Mexico demonstrate the rapid drop in mortality rates that occurred in the 1930s, the period when public health programs began to supplement and upgrade traditional midwifery methods. In 1929 New Mexico had one of the highest infant death rates in the nation with 140.2 infant deaths per 1000 live births. Public health programs were developed in Northern New Mexico during the 1930s[11] and by 1939 the infant death rate had already dropped to 104.3 per 1000 live births and continued to drop during subsequent years. Thus, while the area was still very poor and isolated and had serious health problems as a consequence, the cooperation of the public health personnel with the midwives appears to have significantly increased the chances for infant and maternal survival.[12]

Older health workers in the community have given names of sixteen Anglo women health workers who served in some notable way during the earlier period of public health development and the development of medical clinics. The workers include seven female doctors, four nurses, and five nurse-midwives. Undoubtedly there are other women who were missed, but the list indicates the extent of female involvement in the health care of this area.

Several reasons have been offered to explain the large number of Anglo women healers in this area.[13] Edith Rackley stated, "For one thing, it has been a personal observation of mine that women tend to be in salaried health care positions and men in private positions, and, because of various needs, we had a large number of salaried positions here."

Another contributing factor to the large number of women health workers is that the traditional role of female midwives and other native healers among Hispanic families prepared the way for a greater acceptance of female physicians than male physicians. This was especially true in the area of gynecology and obstetrics.

In addition, many of these women healers went into medicine out of a service orientation, and this was an area of obvious medical need. At times this motive was associated with religious beliefs. For example, Dr. Edith Millican also served as a medical missionary to China, Dr. Mary Waddell was born and grew up in Brazil in a medical missionary family, and the Sisters of Charity were inspired by their religious convictions.

However, this service orientation also was functioning for many of the women who were not working in a program with an explicitly religious background. For example, Jean Egbert, Anne Fox, and Olive Nicklin had been previously associated with similar pioneer work in impoverished areas of Kentucky, and Agnes Walker had done such work in Arkansas.

Finally, a number of areas of medicine, from nursing to the practice of medicine by physicians, were difficult for women of that time to enter. Consequently, it can be assumed that many of the women who did enter these professions were deeply committed to their work and were people who generally responded to a challenge, and people of spirit and courage appear to have responded to the challenge of providing medical care in this part of New Mexico.

It is remembered that these women served with great dedication. Helen O'Brien, current supervising nurse and administrator of San Miguel County Public Health, in a personal interview stated:

It was said that when a nurse arrived in the county, she just took a look around and started working, without even taking time out to unpack. Yes, all the health workers were dedicated people then, working long hours in hard conditions and never missing an opportunity to improve their knowledge. You see, they knew their decisions and skills were so important. In fact, in 1939, New Mexico was one of the top states in the country as far as the education level of our nurses.[14]

Several relatively recent public health developments have had an important influence on the people of the area. One of these, remembered by Jesusita Aragón and the public health workers, demonstrates the extensive cooperation between the public health workers and the traditional midwives.

Before the present large and functional public health building was opened in November, 1963, all the public health personnel and programs functioned out of three small rooms. In fact, the facility was so cramped that the physician would have to go into the rest room with a woman in order to speak privately with her. It was difficult, however, for the staff to get the local politicians to respond to this need for a new building. Finally, in 1960, the midwives in Las Vegas took petitions to their friends and patients throughout the county and obtained enough signatures to force the politicians to respond to the need. When the bond issue necessary to finance the building was finally submitted to a vote, it passed two to one.

Another relatively recent development was the founding of a family planning clinic in 1964 by Dr. Edith Millican. Edith Rackley stated:

Previously, we had never been allowed to assist in any form of family planning. Of course, we all heard of the things distraught women did to keep from having babies, and it just makes your heart sad to hear how desperate they were.

There was so much suffering. It wasn't too unusual to hear of a woman with twenty-three known pregnancies and only a few living children. Their bodies were worn out in childbirth and sometimes they looked just gray. Sad, sad things would happen. For example, a diabetic might deliver a nine or ten pound dead infant then be pregnant again in two or three months.

I remember a very touching story connected with my return to the public health clinic after not working there for a number of years. We had a young woman come to the clinic. She was pregnant with her first baby and had a problem, an Rh factor. She was a young woman and wanted to go to the hospital, but the nurses said, "You are normal, and you can have Jesusita." But the nurses couldn't persuade the girl; she wanted so much to go to the hospital.

They wanted me to talk with her, and I talked with her a little while, and she told me right away. She said that whenever her mother had a baby, the baby died, and the mother would have to go to the state mental hospital. This would happen year after year after year, and the daughter didn't want to be left like that. She wanted to go to the hospital, so the doctor could take care of her and that wouldn't happen to her.

I went out to see her mother who came to the door and said, "My land, Mrs. Rackley, where have you been all these years? I've been having babies one after another and they die, and I've been sick and you haven't been here to help me." You see, she recognized me from the years I had worked there long before.

I said, "Well, now look, we can take care of you; you just come into the clinic," and I gave her an appointment right then and there.

And so the next clinic the mother came in, and Dr. Millican saw her, and she qualified for family planning, so they put her on contraceptives. A few weeks later both she and her husband came back and said, "We've come to thank you," and they had tears in their eyes when they said it. And, you know, when her daughter wasn't afraid anymore, she was able to be delivered by Jesusita, and she had an uncomplicated recovery and a good normal baby.

Many changes have occurred since the 1930s when public health came into this region, and, as previously stated, there was a dramatic drop in infant and maternal mortality in the area. Contributions to this decline include: the introduction of sophisticated pre- and postnatal care, the availability of physicians with modern hospital equipment for complicated cases, an increased awareness among the residents for acquiring health care, and an increased understanding of hygiene and other skills among the traditional, lay midwives.

However, it must also be remembered that important changes have occurred that had little to do with the traditional midwives' skills or lack of skills. Anne Fox, a nurse-midwife who trained local midwives from 1945 to 1964, stated that nutritional education, economic aids, and eventually the introduction of food stamps remarkably improved the general health of many people in the area.

She also stated that when she first arrived in 1945 the impoverished people in this area considered a five to five and a half pound newborn to be good sized, and, by the time she left in 1965, the same group of people considered a seven and a half or an eight pound baby to be a normal, healthy weight. This observation was verified by Jesusita Aragón and several other health care workers. Anne Fox finally remarks that she felt the midwives of this area were especially good at nursing underweight or premature infants along.

During the past few decades an increasing number of

young, private physicians have begun practicing in Las Vegas and the surrounding area, and the style of medical care given has begun to resemble that of the rest of the country. Of the 599 babies born in Las Vegas in 1977, 405 were delivered by male private obstetricians, 40 by male migrant clinic physicians, 98 by a female nurse-midwife, and 55 by Jesusita Aragón, the last of the earlier midwives.[15] Still, the memory of the earlier female health care networks remains, and the consequences of the women's efforts have stayed with the community.

2. Parteras and Médicas

ALL INFORMATION concerning these women was gathered from interviews with older residents in the Las Vegas area.

Maria Aragón. She was from Las Vegas and was born about 1900. She was in the midwife club and took the midwife classes. She gave birth to no children but raised her niece and nephew.

Petra Archuleta. She was from Trujillo and was born about 1870. She retired after Jesusita Aragón started doing deliveries on a regular basis.

Julianita Baca. She was primarily a médica; she only did midwifery when circumstances required her to. She was born about 1843 in the village of Chaperita. Her birth date might be earlier; the records were lost.

Julianita was married at the age of twelve to a man she had not previously met. The marriage was arranged by her parents. After the wedding she moved to the village of San Miguel with her husband. He had to be gone for six months on a buffalo hunt and left Julianita with his mother. Her mother-in-law was hard on her and burned the doll she had brought with her.

When her husband returned Julianita moved into his house with him. The family remembers that he brought an iron stove home with him, the first such stove in the village. At first Julianita was afraid to use it for fear it would melt.

She began having children and had a total of twenty-five, including three sets of twins. Of the twenty-five children only four survived. The family remembers that one child was trampled to death by horses in Julianita's presence and the shock caused her also to lose her unborn child.

She became very ill at one point when she was young and promised God that if she got well she would use her talents to help others because she had learned what it was to suffer.

She recovered and then became a médica but did not deliver babies unless she was really needed. She cured primarily with herbs. Her granddaughter remembers that people would bring gunny sacks of herbs to her, and she would clean and dry the herbs and make powders of them. She kept them in many jars.

People came from all over to see her, from Denver, California, and other places. She especially cured rheumatism with the herb *hediondilla*.

She used prayers and *novenas* to the Sacred Heart to aid in her healing. Everytime she attempted a cure she lighted a candle and prayed to a saint. Her granddaughter remembers that she was very religious and believed her ability to cure was a gift from God. She continued her healing until her death at the age of 105. [This information was supplied by Julianita Baca's granddaughter, Julia Gurulé.]

Carmen Cidio. She is from Las Vegas and was born about 1900. She was in the midwife club and classes and worked for Dr. J. J. Johnson, Sr. She is retired and living in Las Vegas.

Canutita Crespin. She was from Trujillo and was born about 1870. She retired after Jesusita Aragón started doing deliveries on a regular basis. Jesusita then delivered her daughters and daughters-in-law.

Dolores Gallegos (maiden name Córdova). She was originally from the village of Los Alamos and then lived in Trujillo. She was born about 1860, and started delivering babies at the age of eighteen, and stopped about the age of seventy-six. She had learned to be a midwife from her mother, and she, in turn, taught Jesusita Aragón, her granddaughter.

Josefita Gallegos. She was from Las Vegas and was born about 1860. She took the midwife classes and was in the midwife club.

Aurelia Gutiérrez. She was from Las Vegas and was born about 1900. She was in the midwife classes and club and is presently retired and living in Las Vegas.

Gabrielita Lucero. She was from Las Vegas and was born about 1900. She is the sister of Carmen Cidio. She took the midwife classes and was in the midwife club. She is presently retired and living in Las Vegas.

Dona Lujana. She was from Trujillo and was born about 1870. She retired when Jesusita started delivering on a regular basis.

Frances Montana. She was from Las Vegas and was born about 1910. She stopped working as a midwife about the age of forty-two. She has a grown family with two daughters and a son.

Juanita Olivas. She was born in 1897 and lived and worked as a midwife on the Gonzales Ranch, near Ribera, New Mexico. She delivered infants for both her family and others in the area and is presently retired and living on the ranch.

Carmalita Ordones. She was originally from Mexico and was born about 1900. She came to Las Vegas and took the midwife classes and belonged to the midwife club. She had a large family, and her husband was a carpenter.

Simona Ordoniez. She was from Las Vegas and was born about 1895. She took the midwife classes and belonged to the midwife club. People spoke highly of her and she had a good reputation.

Anastacia Ortega. She was from Pecos and was born about 1870 or 1880. She attended the midwife classes and club.

Cipriana Sena. She was from the village of Los Alamos and was born about 1900. She attended the midwife classes and club. She had eighteen children and is presently retired and living in Las Vegas.

Anecita Trujillo. She was from Las Tuces and was born about 1900.

3. Early Female Health Care Givers from Anglo Medical Tradition

INFORMATION CONCERNING these women was gathered from interviews with older health care givers in the Las Vegas area.

Eva Borden. She was a public health nurse-midwife consultant, who worked with Frances Fell and continued the midwife education program in Mora County. (Mora County borders on San Miguel County and shares many of its resources.) She resigned in 1946.

Dr. Sarah Bowen. She came in 1934 to the small facility called Brooklyn Cottage Hospital in Dixon, New Mexico. While there she developed it into Embudo Hospital, which opened in 1940. It became the major medical facility north of Santa Fe at that time and served people from throughout the area, including some from San Miguel County. Using Embudo as a base, Dr. Bowen then developed clinics in the villages of Chamisa, Holman, Chacon, and Truches. She is highly respected and presently retired and living in Las Vegas.

Dr. Nancy Campbell. She was the first obstetrician with the San Miguel County Public Health Department. She was a contemporary of Dr. Sarah Bowen, and, in 1945, she began giving weekly prenatal medical conferences in the El Rito demonstration units. She helped the midwife classes and clubs and went out to the villages when midwives called her for help in complicated cases.

Dr. M. L. Christie. She was born in 1895, took her training in Pennsylvania, and became one of the first Black osteopaths in the country. Her older brother had supported her through school by working as a steward in the Elks Club in Las Vegas, New Mexico, and she came to join him in the late 1920s. She was a tiny woman but very forceful and dynamic and helped to care for several children in the area, providing them with clothes and schooling. She often did not charge people for her medical service and helped people in the area financially. She had a large practice in Las Vegas and was well respected. She died in 1968.

Dr. Hester B. Curtis. She was the director of the Division of Maternal and Child Health in Santa Fe from 1936 to 1941 and, in that position, supervised the San Miguel County nurses.

Jean Egbert. She had previously been with the Frontier Nursing Service in Kentucky. From 1933–34 she was nurse-midwife with the Children's Bureau in New Mexico and demonstrated the benefits of teaching the traditional midwives in Mora County. She made the first true survey of midwives in this area and left written instructions for producing a manual for midwives.

Frances Fell. She was a nurse-midwife consultant from the State Department in Santa Fe. She came in 1936 and resigned in 1946. She did extensive midwife supervision, taught midwife classes, and helped with the midwife clubs.

Anne Fox. She was a nurse-midwife who trained the lay midwives in this area. She had come from England and had worked earlier in London and Kentucky. She began working in San Miguel County in 1946 when Frances Fell resigned. She is currently retired and living in Santa Fe.

Dr. Katharine Gladfilter. She served in the past as head of education and medical work for the National Mission of the Presbyterian Church, which funded and supervised several health care programs in this area. While she was officially in the New York office, she was directly responsible for funding the Mora Valley Clinic and consequently was in New Mexico a great deal. She retired about 1961.

Dr. Mary Lou Hickman. She was the first physician in private practice in Las Vegas who assisted with the Public Health Clinic. She left Las Vegas in 1958. Jesusita Aragón remembers that Dr. Hickman was very helpful to her and gave Jesusita some of her equipment when she left.

Dr. Marian Hotopp. She was director of the Division on Maternal and Child Health, located in Santa Fe. She was instrumental in arranging for the teaching and supervision of the lay midwives and participated in nutritional studies of native, available foods. She resigned in 1953 and, at one point, was regional medical consultant for the Children's Bureau.

Dr. Alvina Looran. She followed Dr. Curtis as director of the Division of Maternal and Child Health. She came to San Miguel County to conduct well child clinics in about 1950 and is currently living in Santa Fe.

Hazel Losseff. She was nursing supervisor in San Miguel County when Helen O'Brien visited the county in 1946. She had previously worked in Eddie County, New Mexico.

Charlotte Maisch. She was head nurse of Embudo Hospital in Dixon, New Mexico, from about 1934 to 1956. In this position she trained the lay midwives. Then in 1957 she was responsible for setting up the San Luis Clinic just across the border in Colorado. She is presently retired and living in Santa Fe.

Dr. Edith Millican. She was born in China in 1914 and received her M.D. from the Women's Medical School in Philadelphia. She first came to New Mexico in 1941 and worked at Embudo Hospital. In 1957 she became medical director of the Mora Valley Medical Unit, and, in 1964, she started a full maternal health program in San Miguel County, including a family planning clinic.

Bessie Moss. She came to San Miguel County in 1934 and was the only public health nurse here until Edith Rackley and the others came in 1936. She went to Albuquerque in the 1940s and later became supervising nurse of Bernalio County.

Olive Nicklin. She came from Canada originally, got nurse-midwife certification in England and worked at the Nurses on Horseback in Kentucky before coming to New Mexico. Edith Rackley states that she identified closely with the lay midwives and was deeply cared for by them. She worked with Jesusita Aragón a number of times.

Helen O'Brien. She was born in 1919, grew up in Boston, and came to San Miguel County in 1958. She is the current nursing supervisor and local administrative head of the San Miguel County Public Health Clinic. She played a major role in forming the clinic as it now is.

Dr. Sarah Pearl. She was the second obstetrician to work with San Miguel County Public Health. She followed Dr. Nancy Campbell in that role.

Edith Rackley. She was born in 1903 in South Texas and received her nursing education at the University of Texas School of Nursing in Galveston, Texas. She came to New Mexico in 1925 and to San Miguel County in 1936 when public health set up a demonstration unit as part of the United States Children's Bureau Demonstration in Maternity and Infancy Care. She became public health supervising nurse in 1938 and received her masters in public health in 1957. She retired in 1965. She has three grown children and lives with her husband John on a ranch in the mountains above Las Vegas.

Dr. Mary Waddell. She was born in 1908 in Brazil and came from a medical missionary family. She became the district health officer for this area and was quite instrumental in the development and building of the modern public health building in Las Vegas. She also worked with Dr. Edith Millican in setting up the family planning clinic and was highly respected by the other public health workers, the midwives, and people in the area. She died in February, 1966.

Agnes Walker. She did pioneer nursing working in Mt. Pleasant, Arkansas, and, in about 1937 she joined Charlotte Maisch and Dr. Sarah Bowen at the Embudo Hospital in Dixon, New Mexico. She died in about 1963.

Notes

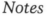

Prologue

1. Clark S. Knowlton, "Changing Spanish-American Villages of Northern New Mexico," in *Introduction to Chicano Studies*, ed. Livie Isauro Duran and H. Russell Bernard (New York, 1973), p. 295.
2. Ibid., p. 296.
3. Ibid., pp. 295–300.
4. Frances Swadesh, *Los Primeros Pobladores: Hispanic Americans of the Ute Frontier* (Notre Dame, Ind., 1974), pp. 201–3.
5. *New Mexico Statistical Abstract, 1977 Edition* (Albuquerque, N.M., 1977), p. 63.
6. *Statistical Abstract of the United States, 1977* (Washington, D.C., 1977), p. 444.
7. According to figures given by the San Miguel County Department of Social Welfare.
8. T. M. Pearce, ed., *New Mexico Place Names: A Geographical Dictionary* (Albuquerque, N.M., 1965), p. 62.
9. Milton Callon, *Las Vegas, New Mexico: The Town That Wouldn't Gamble* (Las Vegas, N.M., 1962).
10. This statement is based on interviews with five older residents of San Miguel County. These five people come from different parts of the area.
11. The village health care tradition in San Miguel County and the surrounding areas was similar in many ways to the traditions described by William Madsen in his book, *The Mexican-Americans of South West Texas* (New York, 1973), which dealt with four communities of Hidalgo County, Texas. His information on this community was originally published in 1959.
12. See appendix 2 for more complete information on Julianita Baca. The information was supplied by her granddaughter.
13. See appendix 1 and appendix 2.

Networks

1. This information is based on interviews with five older, Hispanic residents of the area and five older Anglo public health workers.
2. This information is based on discussions with local people and examination of some public health records.
3. Lynn Perrigo, "The Original Las Vegas, 1835–1935" (Manuscript, 1975), p. 280.
4. Dr. J. J. Johnson, Jr., worked extensively with residents of Las Vegas, and Dr. Kaser aided some of the early public health programs. In addition, some doctors did go out to the people in the rural areas. One example is Dr. William Howe and his wife and assistant Irene who traveled on horseback to the surrounding villages.
5. Lynn Perrigo, "The Original Las Vegas, 1835–1935" (Manuscript, 1975), p. 283.
6. *Ibid.*, p. 427.
7. This information is based on interviews with eight older residents of the area.
8. For more details of the lives of specific midwives see appendix 2.
9. *New Mexico Health Officer, Eleventh Biennial Report, 1939–1940* 9, no. 1 (March 1941): 18.
10. *Ibid.*, p. 27.
11. Myrtle Greenfield, *A History of Public Health in New Mexico* (Albuquerque, N.M., 1962), p. 209.
12. *New Mexico Health Officer, Eleventh Biennial Report, 1939–1940* 9, no. 1 (March 1941): 56.
13. These suggestions were the result of interviews with four of these women. They include one physician, one nurse-midwife, and two nurses.
14. *New Mexico Health Officer, Eleventh Biennial Report, 1939–1940* 9, no. 1 (March 1941): 24 and 25.
15. These statistics were collected by Helen O'Brien, supervising nurse and administrator at San Miguel County Public Health Clinic.

Glossary

adobe a sun-dried building brick made of clay

amigo friend

añil del muerto goldweed, herb for stomach, intestines, yeast infections, and other problems*

arroyos gutters, dry stream beds

atole drink made of cornmeal

azafrán Mexican saffron, a herb used for breaking fevers*

bruja witch

bueys oxen

chicharroñes crisp pieces of meat

Corpus Christi religious festival celebrated with local procession and special honoring of the Eucharist

cuadrilla a dance similar to a square dance

curandera curing woman, a folk healer (curandero if male)

dieta diet, special behaviors for woman for forty days following childbirth

Dios da y Dios quita proverb, The Lord giveth and the Lord taketh away†

Domingo de Ramas Saint Dominic

El que con niños se acuesta, amanece bien mojado proverb, He who sleeps with children wakes up sopping wet†

empacho a stomach disorder believed to be caused by eating too much of certain foods

escoba de la víbora snakeweed or snake broom, herb used for ulcers or to reduce uterine swelling after childbirth*

fiesta celebration

función function, religious festival

hediondilla herb primarily used as poultice for rheumatism *
himnos hymns
immortal a basic remedy used in childbirth and for the heart *
La Historia Sagrada The Sacred Story, a religious book
las manteles del altar the altar cloths
llanos plains
manzanilla chamomile, somewhat like an herbal aspirin, stomach remedy *
mastranzo tea for ulcers
mayordomos managers
médica someone who uses advanced healing techniques, female (médico if male)
mi my
muchacho child, boy
niñas de Maria daughters of Mary
novenas Catholic nine day periods of devotions
Nuestra Señora de Guadalupe Our Lady of Guadalupe, patroness of Mexico
Nuestra Señora de los Dolores Our Lady of Sorrows
partera midwife
patrón protector, leading figure of the village
pazote sweet basil, Mexican tea, used in childbirth as a tea *
procesión procession
romerillo silver sage, wormwood, used in various ways for hemorrhaging, headaches, and other needs *
San Antonio Saint Anthony, a priest and a doctor
San Luis Saint Louis
San Martín Caballero Saint Martin, the horseman or gentleman
San Martín de Porres Saint Martin, Black patron saint of work for interracial justice and harmony
San Ramón Nanato Saint Raymund Nannatus, patron saint of midwives
San Ysidro Spanish peasant who gave freely to the poor, patron saint of farmers and field
santo religious statue of a saint
Santo Niño de Atocha Christ child who gave to those without earthly help, patron of the oppressed
Sierras y Llanos mountains and plains, a community action agency in Las Vegas
tortillas flat, thin cakes
tumbaga gold ring
vaqueros cowboys, herdsmen

vente come

vigas beams

* Information on herbs was found partially in Michael Moore, *Los Remedios de la Gente: A Compilation of Traditional New Mexican Herbal Medicines and Their Use* (Santa Fe, N.M.: n.p., 1977).

† Proverbs from Christine Mather and Fr. Benedicto Cuesta, eds., *Días de Más, Días de Menos* [*Days of Plenty, Days of Want*]*: Spanish Folklife and Art in New Mexico* (Sante Fe, N.M.: Museum of New Mexico, 1976).

Bibliography

Bacigalupa, Andrea. *Santos and Saints' Days*. Santa Fe, N.M.: Sunstone Press, 1972.

Callon, Milton. *Las Vegas, New Mexico: The Town That Wouldn't Gamble*. Las Vegas, N.M.: Las Vegas Publishing Co., 1962.

Clark, Margaret, *Health in the Mexican-American Culture: A Community Study*. Berkeley and Los Angeles: University of California Press, 1959.

Greenfield, Myrtle, *A History of Public Health in New Mexico*. Albuquerque, N.M.: University of New Mexico Press, 1962.

Kelcher, William A. *Maxwell Land Grant*. Santa Fe, N.M.: William Gannon, 1975.

Knowlton, Clark S. "Changing Spanish-American Villages of Northern New Mexico." In *Introduction to Chicano Studies*, edited by Livie Isaro Duran and H. Russell Bernard. New York: Macmillan Publishing Co., 1973.

Madsen, William. *The Mexican-Americans of South West Texas*. 2d ed. New York: Holt, Rinehart and Winston, 1973.

Mather, Christine, and Cuesta, Fr. Benedicto, eds. *Diás de Más, Diás de Menos [Days of Plenty, Days of Want]: Spanish Folklife and Art in New Mexico*. Santa Fe, N.M.: Museum of New Mexico, 1976.

Moore, Michael. *Los Remedios de la Gente: A Compilation of Traditional New Mexican Herbal Medicines and Their Use*. Santa Fe, N.M.: n.p., 1977.

New Mexico Health Officer, Eleventh Biennial Report, 1939–1940 9, no. 1 (March 1941).

New Mexico Statistical Abstract, 1977 Edition. Albuquerque, N.M.: Bureau of Business and Economic Research, University of New Mexico, 1977.

Norwood, Christopher. "Birth Centers: A Humanizing Way to Have a Baby." *Ms. Magazine,* May, 1978, pp. 89–92.

Pearce, T. M., ed. *New Mexico Place Names: A Geographical Dictionary.* Albuquerque, N.M.: University of New Mexico Press, 1965.

Perrigo, Lynn. "The Original Las Vegas, 1835–1935." Manuscript, 1975. Copy on file at Las Vegas Public Library.

Swadesh, Frances. *Los Primeros Pobladores: Hispanic Americans of the Ute Frontier.* Notre Dame, Ind.: University of Notre Dame Press, 1974.

United States Department of Commerce, Bureau of the Census. *Statistical Abstract of the United States, 1977.* 98th ed. Washington, D.C.: Government Printing Office, 1977.